HYSTERICAL CONVERSION REACTIONS

A CLINICAL GUIDE TO DIAGNOSIS AND TREATMENT

NEUROLOGIC ILLNESS:
Diagnosis & Treatment/Vol. 1

Hysterical Conversion Reactions

A CLINICAL GUIDE
TO DIAGNOSIS AND TREATMENT

Michael I. Weintraub
M.D., F.A.C.P.
Clinical Professor of Neurology
New York Medical College

MTP PRESS LIMITED
International Medical Publishers

Published in the UK and Europe by
MTP Press Limited
Falcon House
Lancaster, England

Published in the US by
SPECTRUM PUBLICATIONS, INC.
175-20 Wexford Terrace
Jamaica, N.Y. 11432

Softcover reprint of the hardcover 1st edition 1983

ISBN 978-94-011-6319-4 ISBN 978-94-011-6317-0 (eBook)
DOI 10.1007/978-94-011-6317-0

SERIES PREFACE

Neurologic illness represents a major portion of clinical medicine and challenges the diagnostic and therapeutic acumen of all physicians. It is the purpose of this series to familiarize our colleagues with common clinical disorders and to emphasize not only examination techniques but also to discuss therapeutic and investigative implications. Pitfalls will also be emphasized. In this way, we hope to create a practical set of volumes that will stimulate the reader to "use" these books routinely rather than to set them on the shelf as a reference text.

In the past few years, there has been a revolution in the field of neurology with the development of new techniques for brain imaging and further understanding of the role of neurotransmitters. We hope to meet the needs of our colleagues by this practical clinical series.

MICHAEL I. WEINTRAUB, M.D.
April, 1983

ACKNOWLEDGMENTS

Hysterical conversion reactions (HCR) are among the most common clinical states confronting the physician. Despite the ubiquity of this condition there has been a virtual absence of a standard text on the subject. For over twelve years I have reflected on this topic and have felt the need for a book that would instruct my medical colleagues to deal accurately and effectively with this problem. I was fortunate to work with Dr. Bernard H. Smith who introduced me to the wide spectrum of HCR. Drs. Gilbert H. Glaser and Jonathan Pincus expanded my appreciation of the workings of the temporal lobe and the role of hyperventilation. The above physicians' vast clinical experience and rigorous teachings inspired me to learn more about the "borderlands" between neurology and psychiatry. This interest ultimately culminated in my first monograph: *Hysteria. A Clinical Guide to Diagnosis*, which appeared in the Clinical Symposia series. This had their largest circulation and was subsequently translated into Japanese. The interest generated by this monograph served to stimulate me further into developing a systematic approach to understanding and managing these problems. It is my intention to consolidate the latest information with vast personal experiences into a practical text. I am most grateful to Philip Flagler and CIBA, who have allowed me to reproduce the fine illustrations from our monograph. I also wish to thank *Neurology* for allowing me to reproduce some of the historical plates on hysteria. Dr. Nelson Hendler has also kindly allowed me to publish his useful "Pain form" and Dr. Pierre LeRoy has kindly supplied me with thermographs. I also wish to thank the publisher, Maurice Ancharoff, for his continued support. Most of all I am thankful for the tolerance of my wife and children during this creative effort.

PREFACE

The effects of injury, reactions to life stresses, emotional responses to structural disease, and benefits derived from secondary gain often lead to the development of physical complaints which have no anatomic or physiologic base or are disproportionate to the actual pathology which they accompany. In either case, they often keep the suffering individual from work and prevent him assuming his own responsible social role. The symptoms cover a broad range, extending from blindness through abdominal pain to impotence. They account for untold numbers of office visits, prescriptions, diagnostic procedures, treatments, and days off work. The physician who has not been trained in psychological medicine frequently regards himself as incapable of identifying these disorders by means of behavioral criteria and is often left to guess or conclude by exclusion that a set of symptoms and complaints is hysterical. In other instances he may fail to differentiate their nature and undertake treatment programs which actually add new symptoms to the patient's burden.

It is, however, possible in many instances to detect signs on physical examination or recognize unique features of history that lead the astute physician to the conclusion that the clinical syndrome is in fact hysterical in nature. In order to make this distinction, the challenged physician requires clear ideas about the forms of structural disease, precise knowledge of anatomy and physiology, and skill in the conduct of a physical examination which will identify the signs which characterize hysterical illness. In this volume, Dr. Weintraub lays great stress on his assertion that the symptoms of hysterical conversion reaction may be exhibited by any individual and resemble, though in exaggerated form, the reactions of otherwise well persons to the same stress. He provides a clear discussion of the basic anatomy and physiology from which are derived the techniques of physical examination which lead to recognition of the conversion reaction.

A most difficult problem is the differentiation within the hysterical patient of organic from hysterical manifestations which may be convergent and simultaneous. The majority of patients, for example, who suffer pseudo-angina in fact have coronary artery disease. Two-thirds of the patients who display pseudo-seizures are epileptic. The individual case studies presented in this clinical manual provide systematic and schematized models of clinical study which may help make this differentiation.

Frequently hysterical patients evoke hostility in physicians, who seem to resent them and either make little effort to treat them or decline to do so in the belief that the illnesses are consciously contrived. The distinction between the unconscious behavior of hysteria and the conscious pursuit of primary gain by the admitted malingerer is made clearly. Dr. Weintraub offers a sympathetic and practical approach to the management of the individual patient with an aim toward social rehabilitation. It is here, of course, that the most difficult clinical problem lies, as the patient whose anxiety has been resolved by symptom formation and whose material needs have been met has little motivation for returning to the hassle of daily life.

It is not likely that hysterical conditions will soon disappear, though symptoms reflecting discomfort, dysfunction, disability, and dissatisfaction will assume modified clinical form, reflecting changes in technology and acculturation. Despite the changed clinical expression, the psychic forces remain in common. Hysterical conversion reactions will continue to challenge the physician's diagnostic acumen as well as his capacity for compassionate care. This volume deals with these conditions from a structuralist's point of view.

SIMON HORENSTEIN, M.D.

CONTENTS

1

HISTORICAL BACKGROUND

INTRODUCTION

The origins of hysteria are veiled in obscurity, but one must assume that primitive man was exposed to emotional illness. To him, the world was populated by evil spirits which were responsible for all illness. No distinction was made between physical and mental disease and, therefore, sacrifices, herbs, and prayers were directed toward ridding the body of spirits and demons, thereby assuring survival. These primitive beliefs ultimately evolved into scientific enlightenment and changed with different civilizations and mores. However, vestiges of ignorance prevail today in modern medicine; if we are ever to understand the "mysterious leap of the mind to the body" we must reflect on our medical past. It is not possible to present a comprehensive, detailed history of hysteria within the scope of a single chapter. Thus, trends and patterns of thought will be highlighted so as to give the reader a perspective of evolution of the concepts of hysterical conversion reactions (HCR).

ANTIQUITY

Since antiquity, hysteria has been described as a disease of infinite manifestations and presentations. It is known from various ancient sources that no distinction was initially made between diseases of the body and of the mind. The manifestations of HCR have adapted to the ideas and mores prevalent in each society. Medical knowledge in these ancient and preliterate cultures was integrated with herbal medicine and prayer. Since the development of an illness was considered a curse or punishment for sinful conduct, ritualistic treatment was necessary. Ancient Egypt provides examples of the earliest known thoughts through the discovery of the Medical Papyri. The Kuhan Papyrus (1900 BC), the Edwin Smith Papyrus (1600 BC) and the Ebers Papyrus (1700 BC) all contain detailed references on the concepts of disease. Specifically, a number of strange maladies were ascribed to the wandering of the uterus. For example, "a ball in the throat" was felt to be related to the upward migration of the uterus; fumigation was thought to be beneficial. They did not believe that the uterus was physically dislocated into the throat but rather that it crowded other organs and exerted pressure, producing this sensation. Other complaints such as headache, syncope, and paralysis were treated with pessaries in hope of "luring" the wandering uterus back into place. Specific herbs and incantations were also used. Egyptian medicine thus approached illness as a balance between man and his universe but clearly dominated by the supernatural. It is to the civilization of Ancient Greece that we must look for a refinement of thought and a clearer separation of the supernatural from scientific medicine. Prior to the time of Hippocrates (460–377 BC), an illness was attributed to one disease with variable symptoms. By careful clinical observation, Hippocrates was able to recognize specific disease states with characteristic symptoms. Although he accurately described post-partum psychosis, melancholia, epilepsy, paranoia, etc., and the important role of the brain, he considered disease to result specifically from the interaction of blood, black bile, yellow bile and phlegm — the four humors. In his writings, health was seen as an equilibrium of these humors — whereas illness resulted from imbalance, producing a specific emotional orientation. Hysteria was specifically recognized as a physical affliction exclusively limited to women and caused by a discontented, wandering uterus. He believed that deprivation of sexual relations led to a drying up of the uterus, which, as it lost weight, would wander through the body in search of moisture. Depending on where the organ settled, specific symptoms would arise. The suggested cure was marriage with the practice of sexual intercourse and manipulation of the genitals. The term hysteria itself is a legacy of this period, derived from the Greek word *votepx* (hystera) meaning uterus. Several closely associated Greek words are probably important in sensing the connotation possessed by this term even in ancient Greek times. These are *votepew* signifying failure, inadequacy, or inferiority and *votepos* meaning deficiency and need. Thus, it seems probable that even in ancient times, the term, "hysteria" carried with it a definite connotation of inferiority, failure and deficiency. These words were used interchangeably. The influence of Hippocrates was profound during this time but other Greeks were impressed with the idea that psychological causes could be responsible for physical symptoms such as headache. According to Plato, "Socrates would prescribe no physick for Charmide's headache till he had eased his troubled mind: body and soul must be cured together." Thus, the Greeks were partially successful in separating medicine from magic and religion and there was a serious attempt to place mental illness on a medical basis.

PRE-MODERN

After the fall of the Roman Empire in 476 AD, Europe entered a period of poverty and turmoil which was to last nearly 500 years. During these "Dark Ages" all aspects of arts and sciences declined with a shift away from the physical universe to a spiritual influence. Natural disasters, such as famines, epidemics of disease, earthquakes, etc., helped to further reduce the influence of medicine. Belief in demons as the conveyors of disease and disaster were dominant. In the early Christian era, there was an emphasis on personal responsibility for disease. Sexual factors were primarily singled out. Since demoniacal possession was considered responsible for abnormal mental and physical behavior, exorcism was the cure. Thus, the ignorant populations, representing the great majority, were influenced by the numerous tales of miraculous cures and the saving of persons from the grip of the devil. It was during this time that hysteria ceased to be a specific disease but rather was labeled a mental illness which became the visible token of bewitchment. Books on witchcraft began to appear in the early fifteenth century, contributing to the spread of this belief. The most influential treatise was by Formicarius, published in 1437 by the Dominican Johann Nider, in which detailed sexual activities between women and the devil are detailed. In 1486, the famous guide, *Malleus Maleficareus* (Witch's Hammer) was published by two Dominican Monks for the establishment of the diagnosis and the treatment of witches. This book was so replete with sexual details that it could well be considered a handbook of sexual psychopathology. This publication had the authoritative backing of Pope Innocent VIII and Maximillian I, King of Rome, and led to a fervent search for witches. It became heretical to consider disease as otherwise. This philosophy spread throughout the Christian world and culminated in several celebrated witch trials. It has been stated that this book and the attitudes it generated set back psychiatry for two thousand years. Initially, treatment of bewitchment was kind and supportive but during the sixteenth and seventeenth centuries torture and mass execution were used. This philosophy spread from Europe to the American colonies and culminated in the Salem witch trials. One of the tests for detecting witches was to prick the skin for areas of anesthesia. These anesthetic areas were considered satanic stigmata confirming bewitchment. If the subject did not feel pain from a specific individual known as the "Common Pricker," she was judged a witch. There also existed a spectrum of involvement, and the concept of "temporary" bewitchment was known.

Against this rigid framework, the pendulum of opinion was beginning to sway away from the mystical to the physical universe as a cause for illness. The greatest contribution during this period was made by Johan Weyer (1515–1588) who wrote *De Praestigiius Daemonum* in 1563. In this treatise against demonology, he described his revolutionary handling of a case of alleged fasting. He exposed a ten year old girl, Barbara Kremers, who had won fame because of her claims that she was healthy despite abstention from food or drink. Weyer discovered that the girl's sister Elsa was secretly bringing in her meals and thus her malingering was exposed. He wrote in such a persuasive and easily intelligible style that his philosophy attracted the attention of the educated public. He also distinguished between devilish criminals who should be punished and the vast majority of "witches" whom he considered sick and innocent people. Other attempts to divorce mental illness from theology and ignorance started to appear during this early Renaissance period. Charles Lepois (1563–1633) stated that hysteria was not caused by the uterus but rather originated in the brain and that men could manifest it also. In 1670, Thomas Willis wrote a treatise on hysteria, but it was his contemporary, Thomas Sydenham (1624–1689) who described classical HCR in his *Dissertatio Epistolaris* of 1682. He demonstrated how HCR could simulate every known organic disease in both sexes and in children. Vivid descriptions of convulsive coughing and vomiting, colonic spasms, back pain, and urinary retention were presented.

Searching for new techniques, the eighteenth century came under the influence of Franz Mesmer. In his thesis, *On the Influence of the Planets on the Human Body*, he laid the foundation for future hypnotism and other forms of suggestibility. His pioneering ideas were a mixture of astrology and the current physiology and were known as "animal magnetism." By his use of touch and the hypnotic trance (mesmerism), he was able to produce convulsions, paralysis, anesthesia, and sonambulism. His cures, however, were theatrical spectacles and infuriated his colleagues. In 1842, a surgeon performed an amputation while the patient was in a mesmeric trance. In 1861, a French "magnetizer" came to the United States and cured Mary Baker Eddy of her hysterical paralysis. Thus, for the first time, a really new therapeutic approach appeared, and it could not be easily dismissed despite its theatricality. In France, attempts at refining the diagnosis of hysteria appeared in an 1859 treatise by Briquet. He attributed the hysterical attack to an organic neurosis and described three phases. Modern psychiatrists, in an attempt to restrict the usage of the term hysteria, have used the eponym Briquet's syndrome. I, personally, do not believe this to be correct or valuable and will discuss this later.

Despite the apparent advance in knowledge, it was felt that further exploration of the ability to cure by suggestion was needed. At a research center at Nancy, Bernheim and Liebault collected data on 10,000 hypnotized patients and demonstrated that HCR were due to autosuggestion. They recommended "desuggestion" as the specific treatment.

MODERN

The greatest period of interest came at the end of the nineteenth century when the renowned French neurologist, Charcot, focused medical attention on hysteria in a thorough and systematic fashion. He held his grandrounds at the Salpetriere and demonstrated the entire range of conversions that he believed were of a neurological nature (Plates I, II, III). His position as the greatest physician in France gave the subject of hysteria a dignity that it had never previously enjoyed. Hypnosis was his major therapeutic tool and he proposed that only hysterics could be hypnotized. This belief embroiled him in a major controversy with the Nancy School. Charcot assumed that there was a congenital degeneration of the brain which resulted in a tendency to develop HCR. He did not recognize or ascribe significant psychological conflicts as important in the etiology. He did emphasize their suggestibility and the role of imitation, since his patients were mixed indiscriminately on the neurological wards. Thus, he came to call hysteria the "great imitator."

Since mental illness and especially HCR were considered "organic" diseases of the brain due to specific degenerative lesions, neuro-pathologists and neurophysiologists from all over the world were attracted to Charcot. One was Sigmund Freud and it was not until he became interested in hysteria that the true nature of the condition became known. Few men have been more influential than Freud. His achievements run the entire gamut of psychiatry and his methods and formulations evolved into psychoanalysis. Because his early works dealt with and clarified the etiological basis for HCR, a more detailed description will be provided. During his five month experience with Charcot, Freud was exposed to a wide variety of neurological and hysterical disorders, especially Charcot's hystero-epilepsy. Although well trained in neuropathology, Freud could not confirm Charcot's theory and, consequently, he abandoned the search for a structural defect and instead concentrated primarily on identifying the social and psychological factors that were causative. He became more impressed with subconscious influences on an individual's behavior. From 1887 to 1897 Freud was influenced by the Viennese internist, Joseph Breuer, who, in 1880, had successfully treated a young woman with HCR. This case of "Anna O." became the basis for Freud's collaboration with Breuer and led to the development of the concept of the unconscious and of repression of unacceptable ideas. Briefly, this twenty-one year old woman developed HCR in connection with her caring for her chronically ill father. These included altered speech, paralysis of limbs, loss of bodily sensation, visual changes, contractures, anorexia, and a persistent cough.

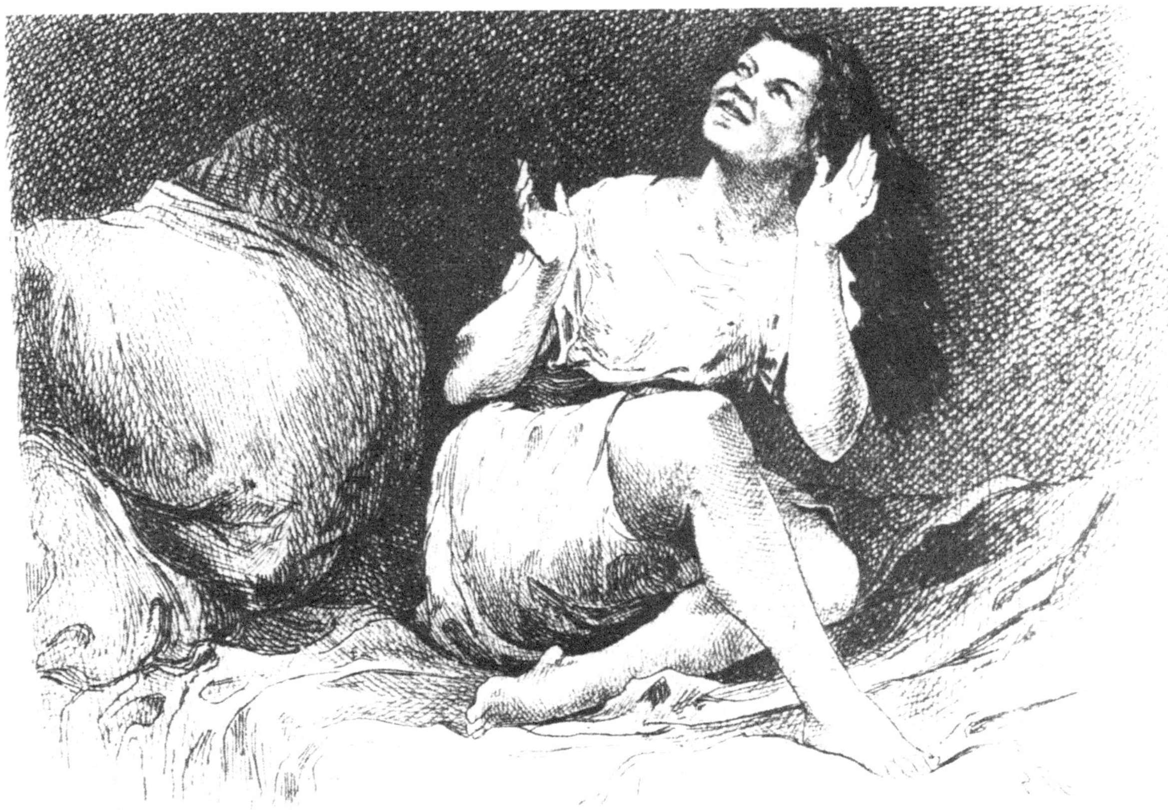

PLATE I. Paul Richer, working in the Salpêtrière was one of the major illustrators in the second half of the nineteenth century. This illustration, taken from his work *Études Cliniques sur la Grande Hystérie ou Hystéro-Épilepsie* (Paris, 1885), is one of a group used to demonstrate the difference between "hysterical" and "real" convulsions and reflected the teachings of Charcot on the subject. (Illustration and caption supplied by *Neurology* and H. Richard Tyler, M.D.)

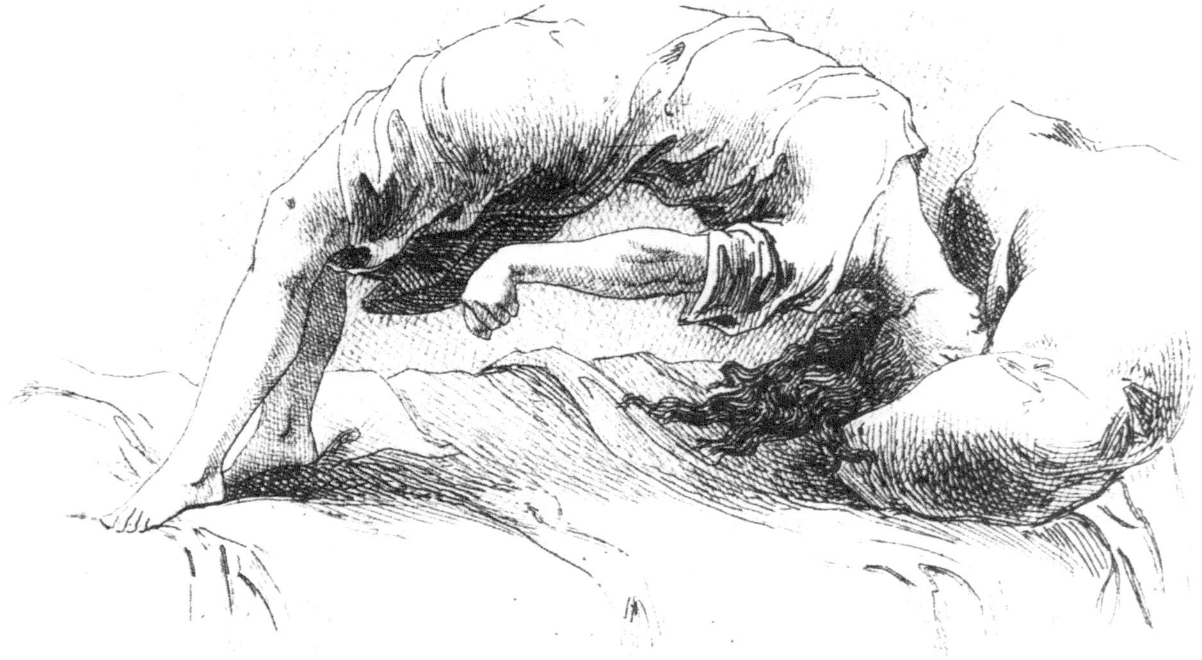

PLATE II. This illustration by Paul Richer, taken from his work *Études Cliniques sur la Grande Hystérie ou Hystéro-Épilepsie* (Paris, 1885), is one of a group used to demonstrate the difference between "hysterical" and "real" convulsions and reflected the teachings of Charcot on the subject. (Illustration and caption supplied by *Neurology* and H. Richard Tyler, M.D.)

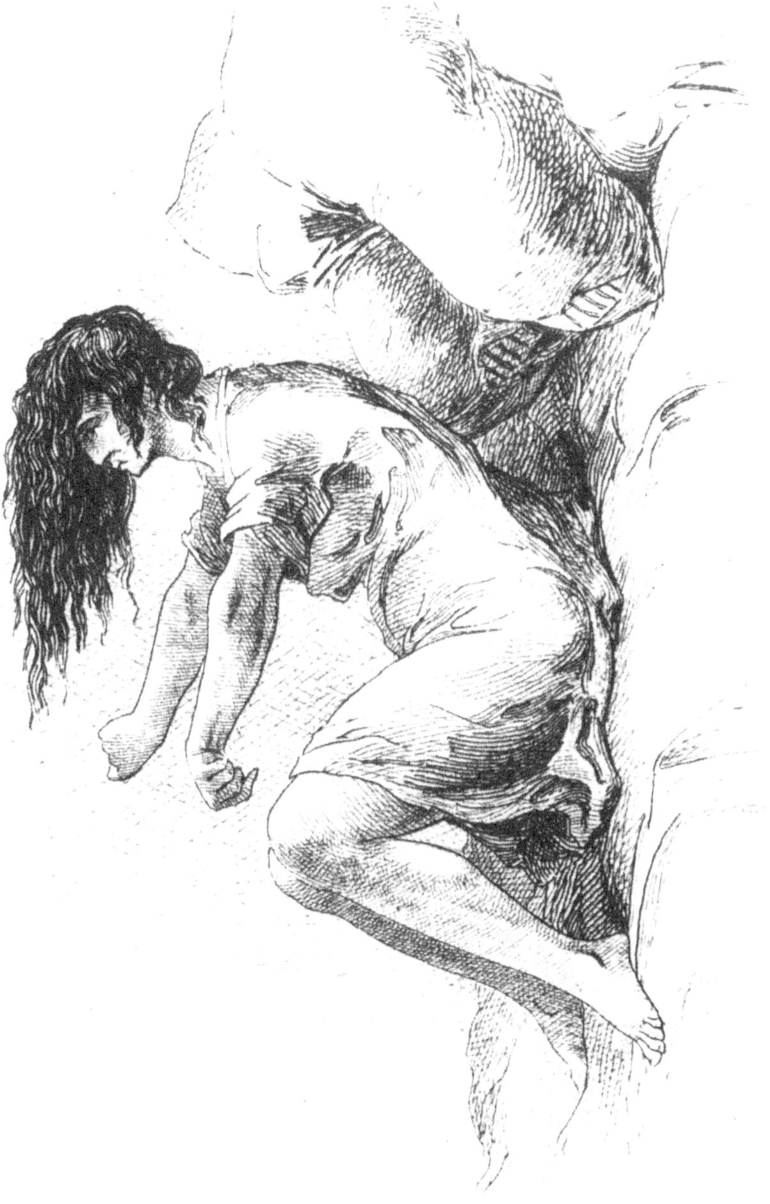

PLATE III. This illustration by Paul Richer, taken from his work *Études Cliniques sur al Grande Hystérie ou Hystéro-Épilepsie* (Paris, 1885), is one of a group used to demonstrate the difference between "hysterical" and "real" convulsions and reflected the teachings of Charcot on the subject. (Illustration and caption supplied by *Neurology* and H. Richard Tyler, M.D.)

Breuer observed that these symptoms would disappear when the patient was able to accept and describe the precipitating event or thought (catharsis). By inducing a hypnotic state, vivid fantasies and intense emotions were recalled, demonstrating ambivalence and sexual conflicts. Ultimately, the latter culminated in an episode of "pseudo-cyesis" as a transference reaction toward Breuer. This case provided Freud with rich material for investigation. In his case of Dora, early symptoms of eneuresis, masturbation and neurosis were present at age eight. By age sixteen, she had experienced isolated attacks of headache, hoarseness, coughing and abdominal pain. By age nineteen, a facial neuralgia was present. Probing into her background disclosed significant childhood memories of her father's illness, sexual affairs, and her seduction by an older man. Freud came to regard these earlier experiences and memories as critically important. As he obtained more data, he became convinced that the early life sexual experiences, real and fantasized, were the basic cause of this future neurosis. In 1893, Freud and Breuer published a "Preliminary Communication" and, in 1895, "Studies on Hysteria" appeared, summarizing their clinical and therapeutic experience. They were impressed with the release of "important memories" by the hypnotic state and felt that the body actively repressed these memories. They noted that transient relief from the symptoms could be obtained in the process of recalling these facts. Thus, they were able to reconstruct a dynamic theory of infantile sexuality outlining several stages of development, i.e., oral, anal and genital.

Failures in development could prevent reaching the mature or genital phase (Resolution of the Oedipal State). Freud held that these early memories evoked intense fear, guilt, conflict and psychic distress and, since they could not be expressed, an active repression process occurred reducing anxiety. This material would become released in a disguised form through the mechanism of conversion. Thus, the psychic conflict is transformed into a physical or mental symptom. The nature and location of the symptom reflects the individual's private symbolism and this type of adaptive maneuver was associated with a primary and secondary gain. The primary gain provided for a reduction of anxiety; the secondary gain allowed the patient to escape from a specific situation. Freud realized that hypnosis was a useful therapeutic tool but it was limited because the repressed events were quickly forgotten after the hypnotic trance. He replaced this technique with the method of "free association," in which the patient is permitted to say anything that comes to mind and, in this way, the unconscious can be probed. By this revolutionary method, the patient could now make a conscious connection between events and symptoms, and this would allow him to "work through" the problem. With this technique, Freud was able to explore and analyze dreams, behavior, slips of the tongue, forgetting, etc., and thus laid the foundation of modern psychiatry and psychotherapy as well as the workings of the mind.

The quest for the cause of neurosis resulted in the most controversial of all Freud's theories, the Libido Theory which included the concept of "infantile sexuality." Freud never attributed to infants and children the complex pattern of adult sexuality. By challenging the innocence of youth, he incurred the wrath of many peers and rigid Viennese society. As Freud became more experienced, he came to realize that actual physical seduction was only a fantasy. Freud and Breuer described two types of hysterical neurosis: conversion and dissociated. The converted symptoms involved the sensory, motor or visual apparatus, whereas the dissociative type produced a splitting of emotions from consciousness. In fact, Pierre Janet, a pupil of Charcot, had previously developed this concept and had popularized the term *"la belle indifference"* to characterize this occurrence. There is little doubt that Freud's theories revolutionized thought and allowed for a better understanding of the HCR. The concepts of conflict between sexual impulses and moral convictions, symbolism, anxiety reduction with primary and secondary gains, etc., prevail today. Freud also believed that males could develop these reactions and, obviously, that the uterus had no definite relation to the symptoms.

Freud's pioneering concepts conflicted with the firmly implanted idea of "innocence of youth" in the rigid Viennese society. Various critics emerged attacking his primary focus on the Oedipal period. Other psychiatrists emphasized the importance of pre-Oedipal conflicts. For example, Marmour pointed out the importance of oral elements in HCR in children, emphasizing cases of vomiting, anorexia, bulemia and globus hystericus. Others attempted to expand the concept of conversion to include a wider range of psychological events that produce emotional conflict.

Adler stressed the importance of sociologic factors and thereby broke with Freud. He advocated short-term therapy. Carl Jung, a contemporary of Freud, asserted that the unconscious material was objective or collective, derived from human experience and had nothing to do with the individual or sexual instincts. Another prominent psychiatrist, Karen Horney, differed from Freud. She emphasized the important role of anxiety in neurosis but concentrated on the importance of the present problem with its sociologic influences. She never denied the importance of past memories and its influence on the patient. Other critics of Freud, such as historian Smith-Rosenberg, in her discussion of hysteria in nineteenth century America, claims that women were playing a social role, resulting from severe regression. Thus, it was the stereotyped female personality who was able to express dissatisfaction with their lives. Revisions and amplifications of Freud's concepts occurred during World War I, when physicians observed HCR ("shell shock") in soldiers who experienced serious threats to life and limb. This term was useful and reduced the stigma of cowardice. It indicated an emotional illness produced by "internal" causes rather than external causes. It also had a patriotic association. It is interesting that when the data was analyzed, a significant majority of patients did not come close to the battlefield or near areas of shelling. Thus it was believed that the presumed threat to life and limb was enough to produce a psychiatric crisis. During World War II similar findings were noted. For example, Abse noted frequent seizures occurring among Indian soldiers between 1942–1945, but rarely occurring among British soldiers during the same period. Numerous psychophysiologic reactions were documented. These occurrences were also documented in Korea and Vietnam. The impact and stress to the personality can be so overwhelming that transient coping difficulties arise. These occurrences challenge the traditional theory of personality development and sexuality as proposed by Freud. Because similar occurrences have been observed during natural disasters, kidnappings, hostage-attempts, etc., we must revise our thoughts about stress and conversion. Because of their increasing occurrence and importance, the DSM III has a special category of post-traumatic stress disorders. Modern day clinicians see this quite frequently in patients who suddenly become victims in auto accidents and develop a "post-traumatic neurosis." I believe this is just an extension of the above coping-mechanism breakdown transiently due to the sudden shock and onset of illness. Individuals from specific cultural backgrounds, or those who are particularly naïve may have a greater predisposition to this "post-traumatic neurosis."

These observations, thus, further strengthen the belief that the precipitating causal anxiety need not be sexual. These conversion reactions clearly offer the hope of escape from intolerable circumstances. Thus, fundamental differences have emerged after Freud's initial concept; presently a combination of sexual, developmental and environmental stresses, all with symbolic overtones, are believed to be important in the development of HCR. The present DSM III has attempted to bring order out of the loosely described terms hysteria and HCR. It is clear that hysteria has remained one of the most important neuropsychiatric disorders, despite all the changes over the seventy five years since Freud's original description.

2

DEFINITION OF TERMS

INTRODUCTION

Over the years, *hysteria, hysterical personality* and *conversion* have been much abused terms. They have been used indiscriminately and interchangeably by the public as well as by the scientific community to the point where they have little value as diagnostic terms. Since the distinction between hysteria and other psychoneurotic disorders is often imprecise and previous attempts to separate them by strict guidelines has been unsuccessful (i.e., DSM I, II, III), it would appear that a new and rational approach is warranted. As can be seen, HCR will not yield to simplistic definitions. Since clinical experience indicates this to be a common medical problem, there is a growing realization that a new and better understanding is necessary if we are to properly treat and understand these individuals.

HYSTERIA

Basic to an understanding of this subject are precise terminology and definitions. At the onset, hysteria should be defined as a class of neurotic disorders which produces *subconscious* alterations of the sensory and motor systems. The dysfunction may be classical and pure, or mixed with other psychiatric or medical conditions. Dissociations of affect may also be present. When these alterations occur, the term *functional* or *conversion reaction* should be applied. This term is to be distinguished from several other usages of the word "hysteria" which have been vague and imprecise:

1. the term used to describe a pattern of behavior exhibited habitually by certain women who are said to be *hysterical personalities* or have hysterical characteristics. This will be discussed in next section.
2. a psychoneurotic disorder characterized by phobias or anxiety, i.e., anxiety hysteria.
3. a particular psychopathological pattern.
4. a term of derogation.

The cardinal features of HCR are that changes in bodily symptoms resemble those of physical disease, i.e., paralysis, anesthesia, blindness, convulsions, headache, etc. — but they have no somatic basis. As we have learned in the preceding chapter regarding Freudian and neo-Freudian formulations, these HCRs provide a defense against extreme anxiety and psychic conflict. There is a transformation or conversion of this adverse psychic energy into physical innervation. The choice of the afflicted region (organ) may be determined by unconscious sexual fantasies or symbolism. In any event, there is a primary and secondary gain by having these symptoms and if these individuals are to be helped, then we must understand the basic precipitating cause and the symbolism.

Traditionally, these disorders occur in young women before age 35. The observed symptoms do not follow known anatomical pathways. Suggestion is quite prominent and is responsible for a great deal of variability. The extent of disability surprisingly does not interfere with the patient's life and survival. Often a lack of concern is evident despite major "body dysfunction," which has been termed *la belle indifference* (Fig. 1). Males can also display HCR but usually they occur in association with financial rewards from trivial injury, threat to life, or under duress, i.e., prison.

It is unlikely that hysterical patients will display all of the "classical" features but the clinician must make allowances for individual variability.

In the DSM II and III, the hysterical disorders were differentiated from the psychophysiologic (somatoform) disorders, which are also induced emotionally. However, physicians have observed clinically that this distinction is not always valid. For the purposes of accuracy and precision, it appears appropriate to discuss separately the psychoneurotic conditions which may cause

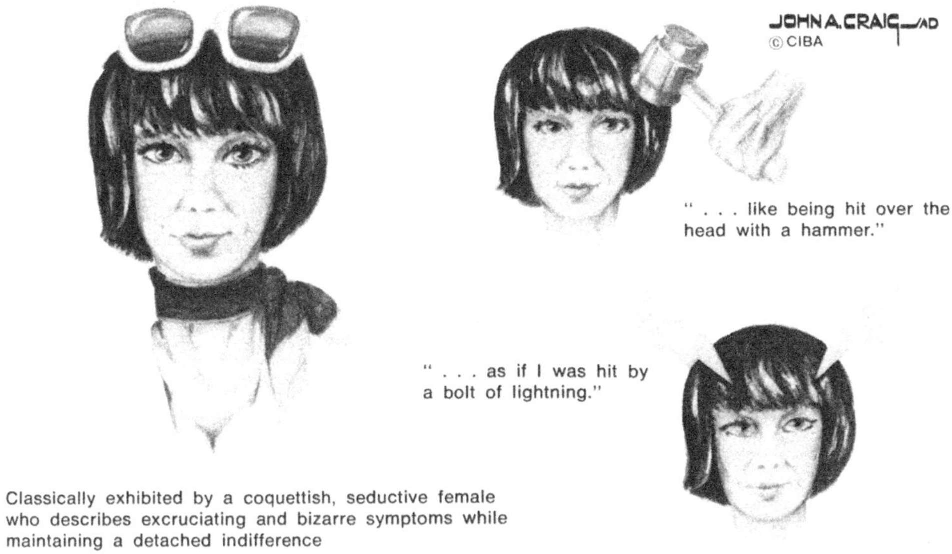

1 "La belle indifference."

confusion. The term psychophysiologic or psychosomatic illness refers to a neurotic disorder arising when anxiety is channelled into the autonomic nervous system. It produces a clinical picture of palpitations, shortness of breath, sweating, diarrhea, blood pressure changes, etc. These somatic reactions are developmentally related to the biological activities that prepare the body for fight or flight (Cannon's Law). They become symptoms when an ambivalent decision is made not to flee, fight or withdraw, while the wish to do so remains. Frequently these reactions have implied a response to fear, anxiety, shame, anger, guilt, sadness, etc. Such expressions are of a *somatic* nature and do not represent psychic compromise or symbolized repressed conflicts, unlike hysteria. I have been impressed with the frequent coexistence of these disorders. These individuals usually have chronic complaints involving multiple organ systems, and have lists of physicians. Some clinicians view these individuals as hypochondriacs. A spectrum of concern may be manifested by these patients to the point of an obsession and phobic fear of a specific illness, e.g., cancerophobia.

MALINGERING

Malingering is another term often used erroneously in an attempt to describe aberrant behavior. This term refers to a *conscious* effort by the patient to deceive in order to obtain a gain (usually financial). Thus, physical and psychological symptoms may be seen. Jones and Llewellyn make the statement that "nothing resembles malingering more than hysteria; nothing resembles hysteria more than malingering." Males predominate with this disorder and in today's society, it most often occurs in association with automobile and industrial accidents. Clearly monetary gain is the primary consideration. Its incidence is *inversely* proportional to the severity of the injury. It tends to be uncommon after severe head trauma and frequent after trivial injuries. Usually these patients have no pre-existing psychoneurotic tendencies. This point has often been used by lawyers in the courtroom as evidence of the sincerity and genuineness of the symptoms; to the sophisticated clinician, there is a contrary interpretation. Having examined large numbers of patients before and after enactment of no-fault automobile legislation, I have been impressed that the number of claims has markedly decreased. The clinician who cares for these individuals notes a *lack* of clinical improvement or change in their symptoms over several months as well as lack of response to various modes of therapy. Objective evidence of damage is lacking. These symptoms tend to appear more frequently among members of lower social and economic groups and financial rewards are the obvious goal. The malingerer deceives others but not himself and his motives are always self-serving, whereas the hysteric deceives herself via unconscious means and seems to be without motive or design. It is obviously extremely difficult to prove the diagnosis of malingering from a medico-legal standpoint unless one can obtain photographs and videotapes or specifically witness the movement of previously "paralyzed limbs", etc. The magnitude and extent of disability from the above described neuroses are immense, especially when one totals its effects on society and the family unit.

It is of interest to note that in a two year followup study of malingering in 50 patients whose claims were unsettled, only two were found to have remained disabled. In nearly all the other patients, the symptoms cleared up *without* treatment, irrespective of the outcome of the claim. Similar disabilities are not encountered in children who sustain identical injuries. Women also tend to have less symptomatology under identical conditions. Even when strongly suspected, malingering is almost impossible to prove and confrontation by the physician is rarely helpful. From a pragmatic and practical point of view, differentiation of hysteria from malingering is an insurmountable task and probably unnecessary. Thus, although the word *hysteria* will be used almost exclusively throughout this monograph, aspects of malingering are implied as well.

MUNCHAUSEN'S SYNDROME

Munchausen's syndrome is a specific subtype of malingering which involves chronic factitious disease. It is infrequent but these patients characteristically travel widely from hospital to hospital, feigning acute and spectacular illness. Hospitalization becomes their main way of life. They willingly submit to extensive workups including invasive medical and surgical procedures. Their medical knowledge is "pseudo-sophisticated" yet plausible enough to fool a significant number of physicians. Dramatic exhibition of body pain is usually the major complaint that often leads to admission. These patients exploit the physician's desire to be helpful, making it almost impossible to make this diagnosis acutely unless one is familiar with the specific patient. These patients often present to the Emergency Room during the "off" hours, i.e., late at night and weekends, when young and often inexperienced house officers are usually in charge. The almost fifty cases described in the literature resemble specific organic emergencies:

1. acute abdominal pain is the most common and is called *laparotomaphilia migans*.
2. sudden hemoptysis and/or hematemesis is called *hemorrhagia histrionica*.
3. syncope, fits and headache is called *neurologica diabolica*.
4. *dermatitis autogenica*.

Irrespective of the presentation, these patients do not respond to any therapy; they show their ambivalence and hostility to physicians, complaining that their condition is worsening due to misdiagnosis and malpractice. Usually the patient discharges himself against medical advice or allows himself to be discovered. The relative infrequency of this dramatic condition has not allowed for a systematic analysis of the psychodynamics but, obviously, the masochistic and psychopathic aspects are significant. One major difference between Munchausen patients and other types of malingerers is that the latter do not leave hospitals prematurely and do not provoke hostility from the physicians. Both of these groups, however, are distinguished from hysterical patients in that they are consciously aware of their symptoms and wish to deceive. It must be emphasized that the presence of a factitious disorder with *acute* physical symptoms does not necessarily imply an absence of organicity. Adhesions and obstruction can occur as a remnant of previous surgery. A poignant example of this was reported by Jensen in which a laparotomy was refused a patient with Munchausen's syndrome, and the patient died from an organic condition. Thus, a thorough workup is always indicated. Since deception is commonly used by drug addicts, schizophrenics, etc., the physician must maintain a high level of suspicion, but this should not overshadow one's clinical judgement.

3

THE HYSTERICAL PERSONALITY

One of the major ambiguities in understanding HCR is the concept of the "hysterical personality". Much has been written to characterize the *typical* hysterical woman, and physicians have come to believe that it is axiomatic to identify HCR by the presence of a hysterical personality. Since the time of Charcot, the personalities of the afflicted have been described. The idea was prevalent that certain personality characteristics evolved as part of the natural history in HCR. This notion is still widely held today and is attested by the large numbers of articles appearing in the literature in which the presence of a hysterical personality is but one of the manifestations of conversion hysteria. I believe this is the greatest source of error leading to confusion about the concept of hysteria. Recently, the APA in DSM III (1980) took a bold and correct position avoiding any reference to personality type as an antecedent condition to HCR. Old habits are hard to break but unless a new approach to understanding is made, it is unlikely that the ancient enigma of hysteria will ever be solved! In order to clear the semantic confusion, a brief look at the background character structure is necessary. In 1958, Chodoff and Lyons described six groups of personality traits which they felt to be characteristic of the so-called "hysterical personality" (Table 1).

Chodoff and Lyons emphasized, however, that these personality traits did not necessarily develop into HCR or dissociative stages. Engel, in 1970, assigned the following traits to these patients:

1. colorful and dramatic expression of language and appearance

TABLE 1.
Common Traits of the Hysterical Personality

1. egocentric, vain, self-indulgent
2. exhibitionistic, dramatic, exaggerated lying
3. emotionally labile, excitable, capricious
4. emotionally shallow, fraudulent affect
5. sexually provocative, coquettish, fearful of sex
6. sexually frigid

2. ability to mimic or play the role of others
3. use of body language for expression
4. demanding dependency in many interpersonal relationships
5. suggestibility
6. manifest sexual problems
7. previous history of conversion symptoms, often starting in childhood
8. other psychiatric symptoms such as phobias, depression, suicide gestures, dissociative states, amnesia and chemical dependence.

Other authors such as Hollender dispute the association of hysterical personality and HCR, indicating that most of these "traits" occur in all women and is essentially a caricature of femininity. This suggests a role play in a male-oriented society. It is of interest to note that several studies have documented a high frequency of passive-aggressive, hypochondriacal, depressive and oral-aggressive traits in these patients. It can only be concluded that personality traits are part of normal; it is only when they become inflexible and maladaptive and disrupt the individual's function that they constitute a personality disorder. DSM III also acknowledges the inherent limitations of reliability of diagnosis since there is a lack of clearcut boundaries separating disorders from normality and there is a significant influence of state and role factors. Thus, most clinicians have come to regard hysteria as an exaggerated form of normal behavior triggered by stress.

LA BELLE INDIFFERENCE

Since the time of Pierre Janet, the term "*la belle indifference*" has been used to characterize the lack of concern of these patients, despite the presence of profound bodily dysfunction (Fig. 1). Over the ensuing years, physicians have come to depend upon the presence of this affect disturbance to help confirm the diagnosis. In my experience, the presence of the classically described "indifference" is not reliably associated with HCR. The reason is that its presence depends on the effectiveness of the personality to repress anxiety-provoking thoughts, and this process may be partial or complete. Additionally, when one is examining compensation and litigation cases with conversion reactions, the practical value of this sign is in doubt because the patients manifest extreme concern for their disabilities rather than indifference. It should also be emphasized that hysterical patients can react appropriately to their disability in much the same ways as normals and patients manifesting psychosomatic illnesses. Rice and Greenfield compared nine patients with *la belle indifference* to normal controls and found no change in heart rate, skin potential or EMG under several experimental conditions.

Thus, it is clear that the terms hysterical or histrionic personality should be abandoned if we are to clearly understand the concept of HCR. These traits are to be considered as exaggerated forms of normal behavior rather than in psychodynamic terms.

4

INCIDENCE OF HYSTERICAL CONVERSION REACTIONS

GENERAL PREVALENCE

It is difficult to write with precision about the incidence and prevalence of HCR because these abused terms have been used to describe diverse clinical syndromes. Hysteria is not a homogeneous entity. While it may be a symptom, it can also be a syndrome due to psychiatric or neurological causes. This results not only in confusion but also in a lack of statistical data. The statement has been made that HCR are no longer commonly encountered by physicians. *This is wrong!* For those of us engaged in the clinical practice of medicine, the frequency and variety of HCR are astonishing. Several studies report figures that range from 5–50%. It is important to note that those with HCR consult all varieties of physicians, but rarely psychiatrists, since they consider their complaints to have a physical origin. The irony is that the overwhelming number of articles about the disorder are written by psychiatrists. Various attempts have been made to classify and quantify (categorize) the range of symptoms seen in clinical practice. While the classical conversions seen in Charcot's time are not seen today, they have been replaced with other symptoms acceptable to the mores of the time. Only by using strict criteria of symptoms and signs that do *not* conform to known anatomical boundaries can true statistics be determined. This diagnosis is *not* made by exclusion and *positive evidence* must be present. Not infrequently, the patient has a specific complaint yet the physician finds on his examination a functional disorder is present in another body area. Consequently, a detailed medical-social history and physical examination are important if the correct diagnosis is to be made.

The natural history of this disease is not always predictable and, consequently, two psychiatrists (Perley and Guze) attempted to establish objective criteria based on the patient's background that would offer accuracy and validity (Table 2). By applying these criteria, the authors felt that a diagnostic accuracy of ninety percent could be achieved. The three criteria are:

A. The patient must have a dramatic or complicated medical history beginning before age thirty five.
B. The patient must admit to twenty five symptoms in nine of ten special review of systems areas (Table 2).
C. No other diagnosis can be made to explain the symptoms.

In their review, these symptoms were scored positive in all ten groups when they caused the patient to see a physician or to take medication or if the symptom interfered with the patient's life to a significant degree. It is of interest that areas 2 and 8 of the review are unusually positive. This finding suggested to them that a useful screen for hysteria would be to ask questions about sexual problems and conversion alone. Woodruff feels quite strongly that if the history is reliable and there are no symptoms in areas 2 and 8, then the diagnosis of hysteria, using the Perley-Guze criteria is not possible. I do not believe this statement to be true and it is contrary to my clinical experience and the experience of many of my colleagues. It should be noted that one-third of the symptoms of area 2 were not explained and, therefore, it is dangerous to make the diagnosis of hysteria on the basis of unexplained neurological symptoms. This point has been emphasized by Slater and more recently by Weintraub. In addition, a diagnosis of hyperventilation syndrome could cause 18 of the symptoms found in seven of their ten categories (Pincus & Tucker).

The concept of HCR has essentially excluded men and been considered a female disease. Previous statistics by Luisada *et al.* found an occurrence of 1/1,000 males with the diagnosis of HCR. Arkonac and Guze estimated the prevalence rate to be one to two percent of the female population. It has also been recognized in family studies that there is a tenfold increase in incidence among first degree female relatives of a woman with HCR. When a male developed HCR, it was expected that he would show feminine traits and a typical hysterical personality. This was described in

TABLE 2.
Perley and Guze Criteria for Retrospective Diagnosis of Hysteria

Group 1	Headaches Sickly most of life
Group 2	Blindness Paralysis Anesthesia Aphonia Fits or convulsions Unconsciousness Amnesia Deafness Hallucinations Urinary retention Ataxia Other conversion symptoms
Group 3	Fatigue Lump in throat Fainting spells Visual blurring Weakness Dysuria
Group 4	Breathing difficulty Palpitation Anxiety attacks Chest pain Dizziness
Group 5	Anorexia Weight loss Marked fluctuations in weight Nausea Abdominal bloating Food intolerances Diarrhea Constipation
Group 6	Abdominal pain Vomiting
Group 7	Dysmenorrhea Menstrual irregularity, including amenorrhea for at least two months Excessive menstrual bleeding
Group 8	Sexual indifference Frigidity Dyspareunia Other sexual difficulties Vomiting for all nine months of pregnancy or hospitalized for hyperemesis gravidarum
Group 9	Back pain Joint pain Extremity pain Burning pains of sexual organs, mouth or rectum Other bodily pains
Group 10	Nervousness Fears Depressed feelings Need to quit working or inability to carry on regular duties because of feeling sick Crying easily Feeling life was hopeless Thinking a good deal about dying Wanting to die Thinking of suicide Suicide attempts

1859 when Paul Briquet reported 430 cases of hysteria with seven appearing in males. These patients were caricatures of femininity and felt to be passive homosexuals. By 1886, the diagnosis of male hysteria was increasing and changing in concept especially in England due to the rising incidence of "railway spine" (Page & Putnam).

A specific type of HCR has been described in males called the Ganser syndrome. This is a controversial entity occurring in male prisoners in which approximate answers (paralogic responses) are given. Further characterization of this disorder includes sudden onset and termination, short duration of symptoms, temporary clouding of consciousness with paralogic responses, absence of malingering. Recently, Fuente *et al.* emphasized an association with previous head trauma, onset of symptoms after release from confinement and absence of premorbid psychotic illness. The symptoms all resolve spontaneously with subsequent amnesia. I recently noted this syndrome to occur in a 15-year old boy who took his father's car while under the influence of alcohol. He did not have a license and the car was involved in a serious accident. He was brought by ambulance to the hospital whereupon examination gave approximate answers about his identity yet could cooperate in most other areas with accurate information. Fear, embarrassment and guilt were major factors in precipitating these symptoms. Within ten hours, all approximate answers disappeared with amnesia for the event.

CULTURAL ASPECTS

Clinicians must be aware of *cultural concepts of illness*. Due to the increasing ethnic diversity of our population, many clinical presentations are acceptable. For example, in 1969, Finney described the high incidence of HCR in Appalachian males, who, brought up under the Puritan work ethic, found a culturally acceptable "way out" after they lost their jobs and could not support their families. He felt that poverty and ignorance were significant factors. In Hispanic Hysteria or the "Puerto Rican syndrome" both men and women present with "ataques" of possession by spirits. They manifest mutism, inability to eat and pseudoepileptic fits which are acceptable responses within the spiritualistic culture. These episodes may last minutes to hours depending on the significance of the secondary gain. In those populations with more African ties, Voodism is important and this can be seen in the report of Hillard and Rockwell. This is not infrequent in the Southern USA, where there is a "hexing" culture and "Rootism," where the symptoms can only be cured by lay practitioners or "Root doctors." Many investigators believe that HCR are restricted to uneducated, primitive and unsophisticated individuals who present with various symptoms depending on their concepts of illness (physical). This is not supported by clinical observation. Given adequate stress, there is no reason to believe that anyone is immune. It is true, however, that such groups are more likely to display bizarre and spectacular HCR, whereas the more sophisticated patients will manifest symptoms consonant with prevailing concepts of illness.

EPIDEMIC HYSTERIA

Cultural, physical and emotional factors play a significant role in epidemic hysteria. Worldwide occurrences have been reported with over 37 specific incidents since 1900. Schools and work environments provide appropriate settings. In 1979 the *British Medical Journal* reported that 196 Jamaican children suddenly developed abdominal pains, vomiting, diarrhea, fainting and hyperventilation. None of the teachers or parents became ill and organic causes were ruled out. This outbreak shared many common features with previous epidemics suggesting that the diagnosis of hysteria be strongly considered if: 1) girls make up 70–100% of those affected, 2) ages 12–14 are usually first involved followed by younger groups, 3) waves of involvement occur, 4) family members and teachers are healthy, 5) subjective complaints are exaggerated in the absence of physical findings.

Marching bands are another group that seems predisposed to these epidemics. On October 16, 1980 22 members of the Alabama Carver High School band were hospitalized after fainting, coughing, nausea and chest pains at a football game. Dr. Michael Levine reported in *JAMA* on another Alabama high school marching band whose members developed mass hysteria at halftime ceremonies during a football game. He believes that two preconditions are necessary in order to have such a contagious and mass effect: 1) a general state of tension, and 2) a relevance of the behavior to the situation being experienced by others.

While these epidemics are alarming, all organic possibilities must be entertained and ruled out. These outbreaks are usually prolonged and extended, due to the anxiety generated in parents, health officials, police, press, etc. Firm reassurance, as soon as possible, may be successful. If this does not work then each individual should be quickly separated from the group; by dividing the individuals, the epidemic will be conquered. (Forrester, RM) This policy was also advocated as early as the sixteenth century by Johan Weyer. Thus social and environmental pressures are significant factors.

In summary, it is clear that the symptoms a person manifests are derived from a complex interaction of intrapsychic conflicts, cultural patterns, environment and concepts of illness. Emotional immaturity and dependency factors are more important than socio-economic and educational level. HCR can occur in any person at any point in time, depending on the circumstances.

Before we discuss clinical manifestations a word about history taking. Interview techniques are not as thoroughly developed by physicians due to time pressures, etc. The usual medical history consists of a description of the chief complaint followed by a detailed description of the present illness.

A good history is critical. Interview techniques have not been thoroughly developed by physicians due to the limitations of time and the urgency of an "organic presentation." In addition, the increased reliance on the laboratory for diagnosis has created short cuts. A thorough medical history will allow the physician to accurately arrive at the correct diagnosis 80–90% of the time. It is thus important to develop interviewing techniques that will identify past medical facts, social, work and litigation factors as well as family history — that will provide clues to the diagnosis. By such a meticulous process it will become clear how the individual perceives the illness, as well as the basic psychodynamics and coping patterns. The general level of maturity will also be noted and become important when the choice of a therapy is considered. Elsewhere, we discuss the Perley-Guze criteria for historical documentation; these data suggest risk factors. A history of multiple surgical procedures suggests poor coping and poor prognosis. Another important aspect of the past medical history is whether the patient has ever observed other individuals (in person or on television) with the same symptom(s). Since subconscious influences are present, the history may not be totally accurate. Personal habits should be questioned: the excessive use of alcohol or cigarettes may be a partially successful means of anxiety control.

Familial occurrence of HCR is seen in at least 20% of individuals and imitation and organ response are frequently seen in females. Environmental factors and similar religious beliefs are common.

The physical examination is the next step in the systematic evaluation of the patient. Entire textbooks have been written describing the methods to be employed; in this chapter we will highlight the major aspects. Since the finding of *positive* signs on the physical examination is the keystone to correct diagnosis, it is important to be very thorough. Often it will be necessary to perform serial testing to establish the diagnosis. The patient should be observed in removing garments of clothing — not only to determine how the extremities move and the presence of subtle associative movements: aspects of the patient's basic personality are demonstrated by his reaction to his own body and the physician's examination of it. The physician should avoid embarrassing the patient and the patient's comfort should always be maintained. Inspection of the body will identify scars, birth marks, scoliosis and deformities that might not have been noticed before. This might escape notice during "emergency" evaluations for an alleged organic condition, but the physician must be thorough, as it may help in diagnosis.

5

CRITERIA FOR DIAGNOSIS ON PHYSICAL EXAMINATION: Basic Principles of Anatomy and Physiology

The most important point to remember in recognizing and treating the hysterical patient is that the diagnosis is *not* made by exclusion. There must be *positive* evidence demonstrating that the dysfunction is functional in origin rather than organic. *It is not a diagnosis of exclusion*. Because most bodily dysfunction is in the neurological area, the neurologist, by dint of his expertise in neuroanatomy and neurophysiology, is best equipped to diagnose modern day HCR by showing inconsistencies on examination. It is only with the presence of such inconsistencies and their ability to change with suggestion that one can accurately arrive at the correct diagnosis. The application of the Perley-Guze criteria is an important part of the historical documentation that supports the clinical diagnosis. The following section will review basic neuroanatomic and physiologic principles that will allow the physician to feel more comfortable in diagnosis and management.

Possibly no part of the neurological examination is more frequently involved and more difficult to evaluate than the testing of sensation. The clues to hysterical sensory loss are its failure to conform to anatomic and physiologic patterns of innervation, and the variations that occur on multiple examinations with suggestion. Since sensory testing is difficult for both the patient and the clinician, it is desirable to keep the number of tests to a minimum and at the same time to choose the simplest and the most reliable

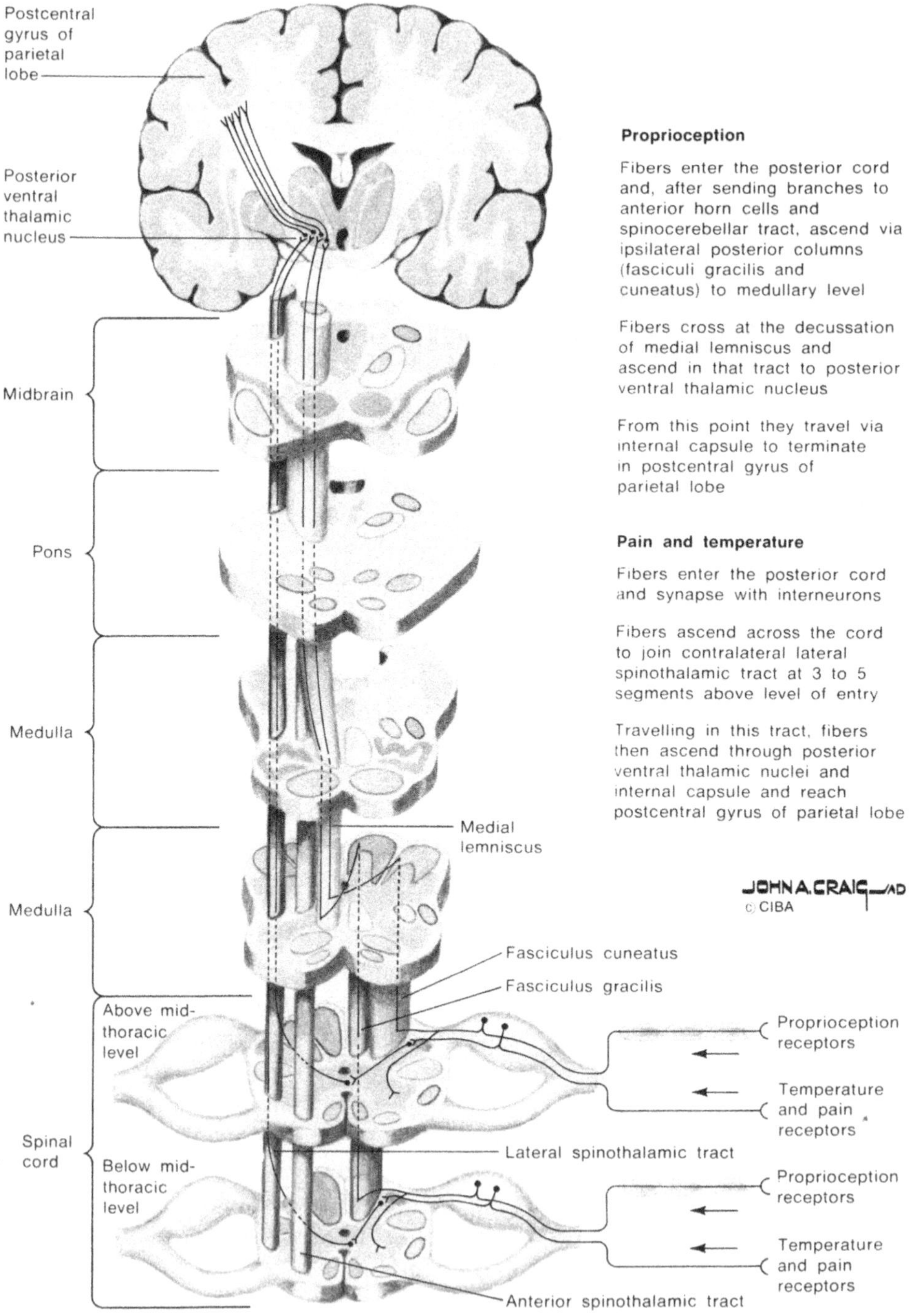
Postcentral gyrus of parietal lobe
Posterior ventral thalamic nucleus
Proprioception
Fibers enter the posterior cord and, after sending branches to anterior horn cells and spinocerebellar tract, ascend via ipsilateral posterior columns (fasciculi gracilis and cuneatus) to medullary level
Fibers cross at the decussation of medial lemniscus and ascend in that tract to posterior ventral thalamic nucleus
From this point they travel via internal capsule to terminate in postcentral gyrus of parietal lobe
Pain and temperature
Fibers enter the posterior cord and synapse with interneurons
Fibers ascend across the cord to join contralateral lateral spinothalamic tract at 3 to 5 segments above level of entry
Travelling in this tract, fibers then ascend through posterior ventral thalamic nuclei and internal capsule and reach postcentral gyrus of parietal lobe
Midbrain
Pons
Medulla
Medial lemniscus
Medulla
JOHN A. CRAIG AD
© CIBA
Fasciculus cuneatus
Fasciculus gracilis
Above mid-thoracic level
Proprioception receptors
Temperature and pain receptors
Spinal cord
Lateral spinothalamic tract
Below mid-thoracic level
Proprioception receptors
Temperature and pain receptors
Anterior spinothalamic tract

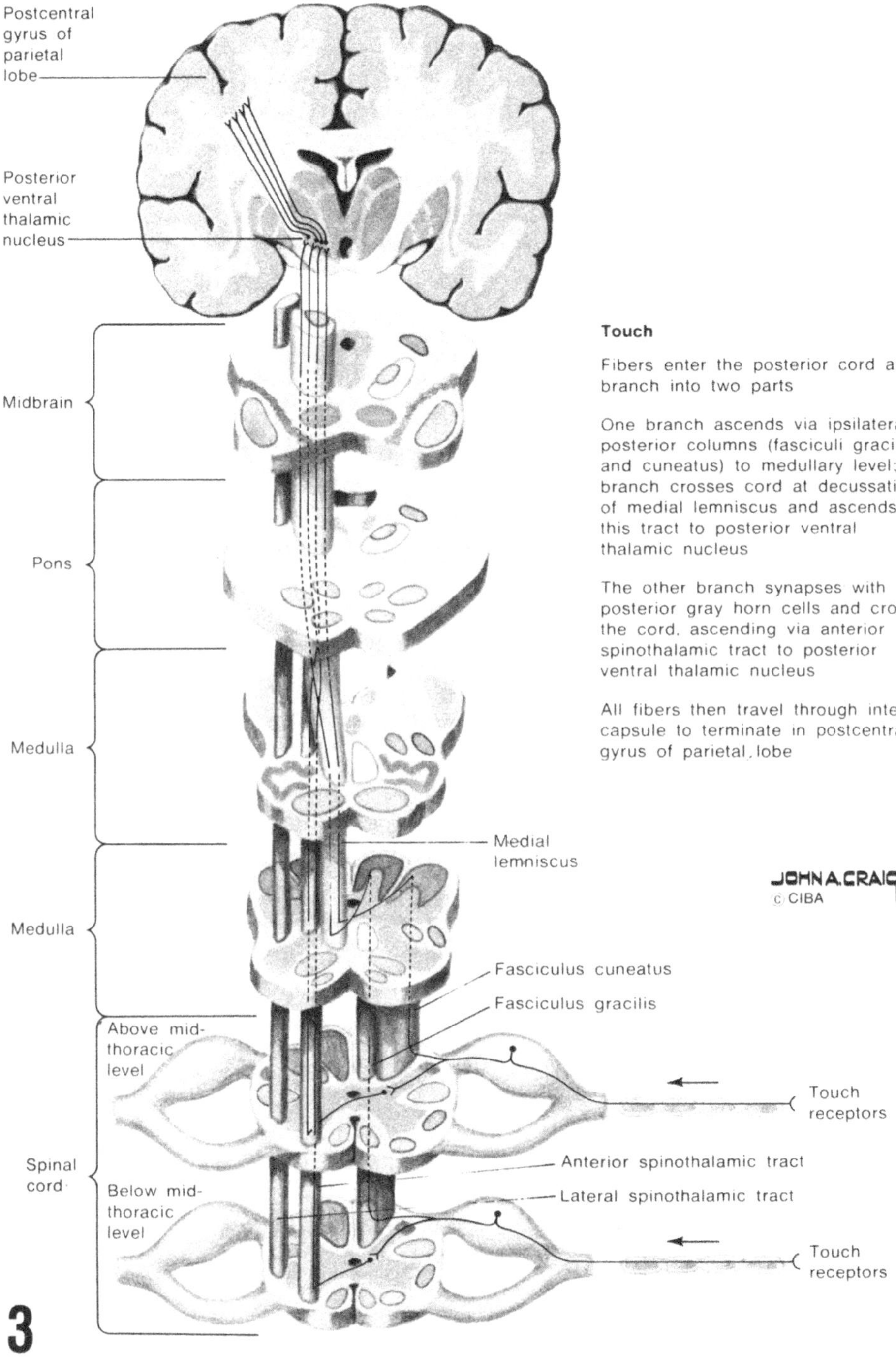

Touch

Fibers enter the posterior cord and branch into two parts

One branch ascends via ipsilateral posterior columns (fasciculi gracilis and cuneatus) to medullary level; branch crosses cord at decussation of medial lemniscus and ascends in this tract to posterior ventral thalamic nucleus

The other branch synapses with posterior gray horn cells and crosses the cord, ascending via anterior spinothalamic tract to posterior ventral thalamic nucleus

All fibers then travel through internal capsule to terminate in postcentral gyrus of parietal lobe

3

Ascending tracts (Figures 2 and 3).

tests. The three sensory modalities of position, light touch and pain-temperature appreciation offer the best results in the determination of evaluation of sensory status. Peripheral sensory receptors have been classified according to the information they convey. Different pathways exist which allow the human organism to consciously experience these sensations. The sensory system is somewhat more complicated than the motor system since it has two long tracts on each side of the spinal cord (Fig. 2).

One of these contains *proprioceptive fibers*, which pass in the posterior root to the posterior column and then stay ipsilateral up to the level of the medulla. At this level there is a decussation of fibers to form the medial leminiscus which ascends to relay in the posterior ventral nucleus of the thalamus. The fibers then continue to the postcentral gyrus and parietal lobe for conscious appreciation. The other major tract carries *pain-temperature sensations* from the periphery, through the dorsal root and across the central canal of the spinal cord to form the lateral spinothalamic tract (LST). This crossing is obliquely upwards and forward with the fibers reaching the opposite side three-five segments higher than the body segments they subserve. This important anatomical fact has clinical significance. The fibers in the LST then ascend to the posterior ventral nucleus of the thalamus, but from this point their further pathway is unknown.

Light touch is another sensation arising in the periphery that travels through the spinal cord by two ascending pathways (Fig. 3). One path is via the ipsilateral posterior column and the other is via the contralateral ventral spinothalamic tract (VST). Thus this double representation accounts for touch preservation in serious organic spinal cord lesions. Thus, when the clinician is confronted with a patient manifesting absence of touch perception, he must expect to see extensive myelopathy or a patient with a functional disorder.

Vibration appreciation is another sensation that has clinical use. It has been theorized that this sensation is carried by two fiber tracts; one arising and travelling with the pyramidal tract, and the other travelling in the ipsilateral posterior columns. Very frequently patients lose vibration sense over unilateral bony areas; this is a noteworthy clinical observation helping to confirm the diagnosis of HCR when an intact bony skeleton can be demonstrated.

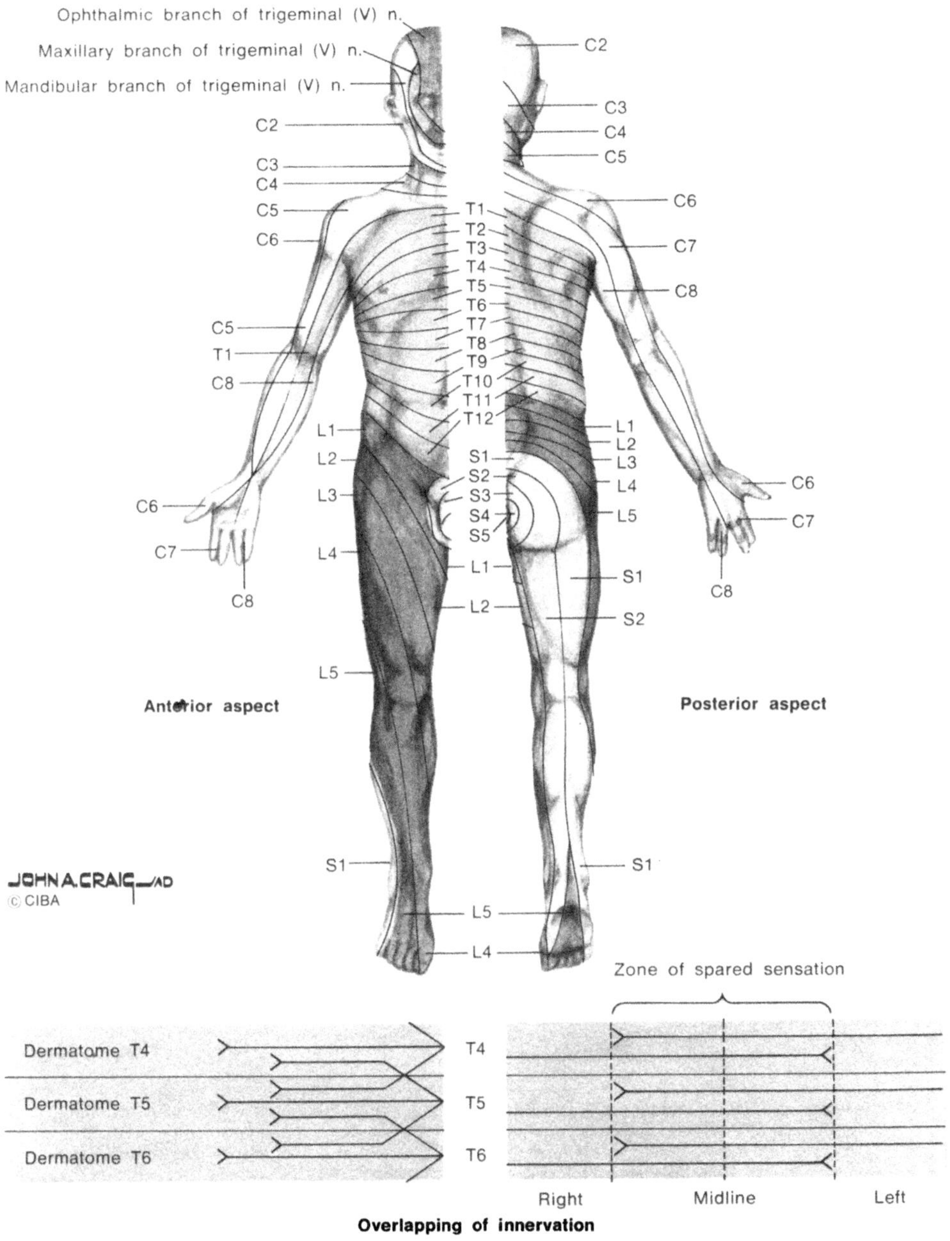

Considerable overlapping of the nerve supplies of adjacent dermatomes accounts for sensory sparing if only a single root is injured

Overlapping of innervation from right and left sides creates zone of spared sensation at anterior midline in unilateral injury

4 Cutaneous distribution of spinal dermatomes (after Keegan).

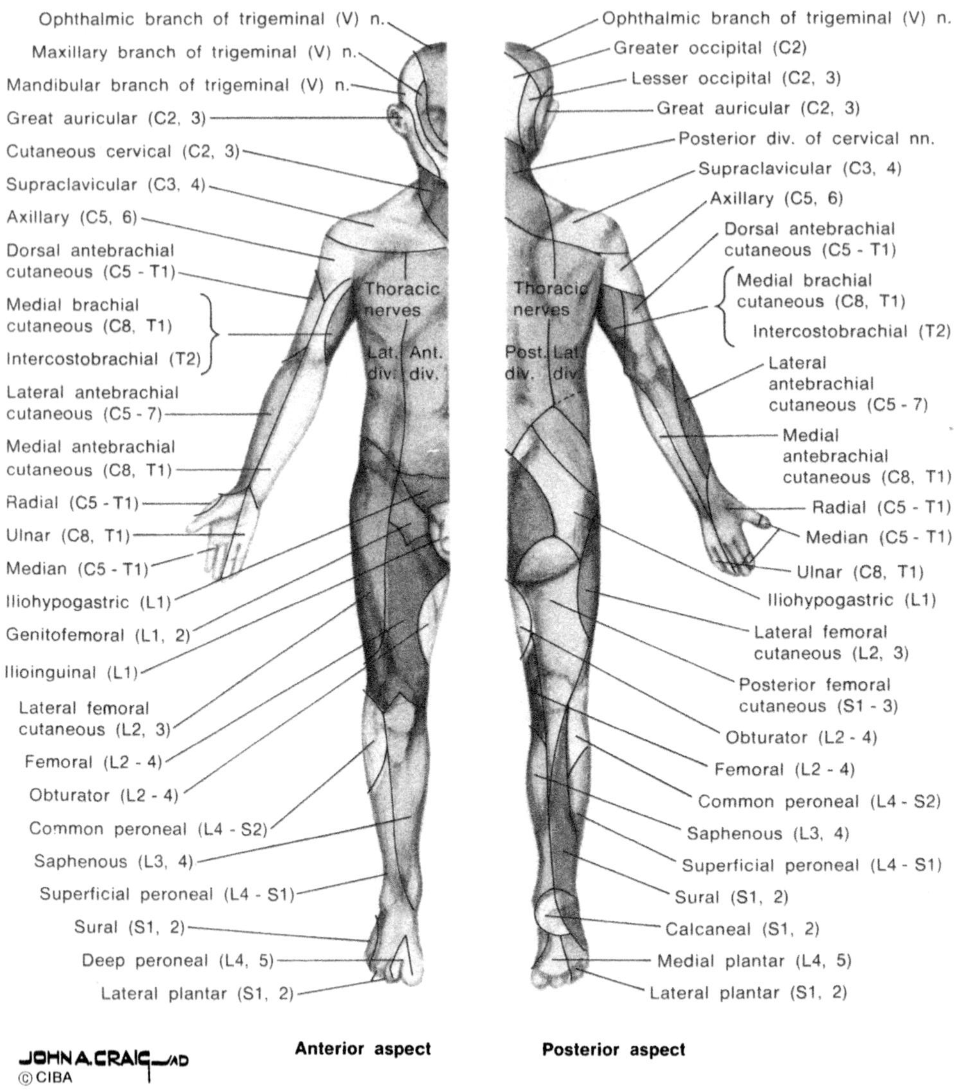

Loss of sensory modalities is based on the anatomic location of the inciting lesion. The pattern of loss may follow either a spinal dermatome pattern or one based on peripheral nerve damage. Because exact peripheral nerve distribution varies among individuals, patterns may differ

Note that isolated islands of anesthesia (*e.g.*, axillary and deep peroneal) can exist on an anatomic basis

5 Cutaneous distribution of peripheral nerves (after DeJong).

With this basic anatomical knowledge of the sensory pathways one can more readily approach and understand bizarre sensory patterns and symptoms. It should be stated that disturbances of skin sensation may occur in any location, shape and pattern, but they most often follow skin surface concepts of body division rather than neurological patterns of sensation (Figs. 4, 5). As seen from Table 3, these symptoms not only fail to conform to known anatomy and physiology, but the findings also change on multiple examinations and with suggestion. There are four major categories of sensory alteration: 1. anesthesia, 2. hypesthesia, 3. dysesthesia, and 4. hyperpathia. These may be the essential features of the complaint, or may be discovered incidentally in the course of the examination. They may be an isolated finding, or co-exist with motor abnormalities. Their onset can be sudden and dramatic and may last a variable period of time. The pattern usually changes with repeated examinations and suggestibility.

TABLE 3. Hysterical Sensory Patterns

1. Failure to conform to anatomic and physiologic patterns.
2. Changing results on multiple examinations.
3. Pattern changes with suggestion.

6

CLINICAL PRESENTATIONS IN ADULTS

SENSORY DISTURBANCES

I have found the following observations especially helpful although not infallible in trying to distinguish hysteria from organic disease. In the case of hysterical anesthesia the lack of sensation is much more extensive than that seen in organic lesions and tends to involve *all* sensory modalities. (Fig. 6) The margins are more sharply defined into the so-called stocking-glove pattern with absolute borders ending at joints, skin-creases or the midline. Most patients are unaware that in organic sensory loss there is para-median sparing due to the interdigitations of the peripheral nerve endings. There are also gradual borders in the joints for the same reasons. Commonly an extremity on one side of the body becomes involved and this is usually the *dominant* one for the patient. In hysterical hemianesthesia there is often a loss of vision and hearing ipsilaterally. Commonly there is a dense sensory loss down the front of the body (anterior) with *sparing* of the back (dorsal). In addition, if vibration is tested over the frontal bone, sternum or ribs, patients invariably state that the "diseased side" is less responsive. They are unaware that bone conduction is being tested in these instances.

Case: Recently a 24 year old immature female was struck in the face during a bar-room fight. She complained of total loss of sensation over the involved side of the face as well as the body. She also lost her ability to smell. Examination confirmed functional

Demarcation

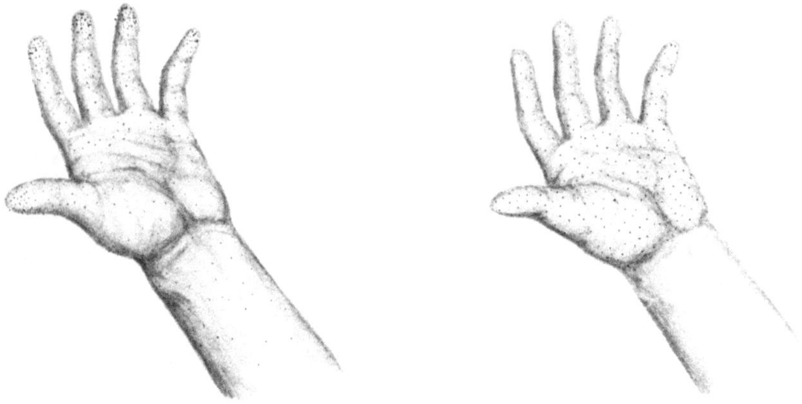

A. Organic (*e.g.*, polyneuritis): sensory loss more profound distally; gradual transition to area of normal sensation

B. Hysterical: sensory loss uniform; sharp demarcation from area of normal sensation, usually at external anatomic landmark (*e.g.*, joint, skin fold) rather than along a nerve distribution

JOHN A. CRAIG AD
c CIBA

Dissociation

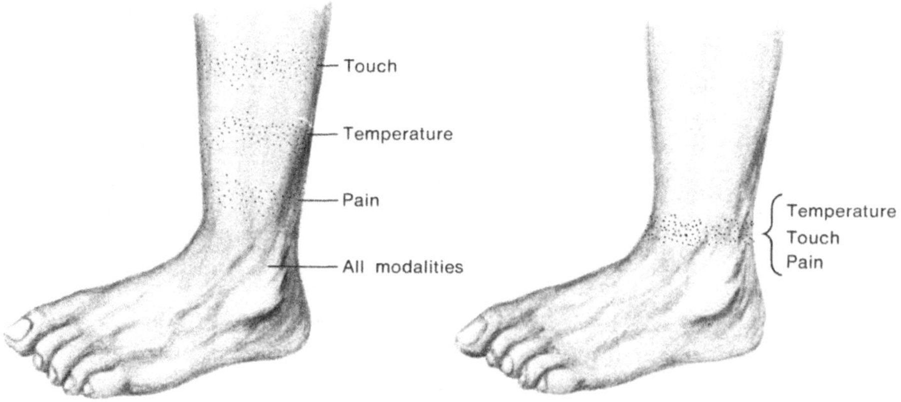

A. Organic: different level of loss for each sensory modality

B. Hysterical: single level of loss for all sensory modalities

6 Stocking-glove anesthesia.

sensory loss and functional loss of smell (ammonia test). Trigeminal nerve function and corneal reflexes were intact.

Hyperventilation is perhaps the most common cause for sensory complaints and the physician can reproduce the patient's symptoms by this maneuver. Overbreathing is the most common response to anxiety and young females 15–35 years old appear to be most susceptible. A variety of complaints are described, including headache, dizziness, sweating, syncope, nausea-vomiting, paresthesiae of lips and fingers, and these can be reproduced by the clinician by asking the patient to voluntarily overventilate.. In just four minutes of hyperventilation, the cerebral blood flow can be reduced by 40% resulting in cerebral hypoxia and slowing on EEG (Plum & Posner). The hyperventilation response is not only seen in hysterical patients but in all the anxiety neuroses, i.e. hypochondriasis, psychosomatic disease, etc. It is not surprising that in a study of 500 consecutive patients seen by a gastroenterologist, frequencies of 76, 60 and 55% were seen for shortness of breath, palpitations and chest pain respectively (McKell & Sullivan). In a neurological population Pincus found that 77% of patients with Hyperventilation (HV) syndrome had a history of previous psychosomatic illness and that females 15–45 years old were most susceptible. Psychogenic head pain may also provoke a HV response. The clinician should use the HV maneuver in his examination in an attempt to reproduce the patient's symptoms or witness bizarre "spells."

Polyneuropathy secondary to diabetes mellitis, uremia, alcoholism, toxins, etc., characteristically affect the most distal portions of the extremities in a symmetrical fashion and may produce subjective numbness and tingling of the digits. A glove-stocking sensory deficit with gradual borders is encountered. However, hysterics tend to demonstrate absolute borders with complete analgesia-anesthesia to all modalities. This is an anatomic impossibility especially if it arises in one extremity *without* motor or reflex changes. Additionally, an EMG with sensory and motor conduction velocities and H-reflex analysis will indicate if there are any objective elements present.

The vibrating tuning fork (128 cps) is a useful instrument for the clinician and will help him to clarify difficult sensory patterns. If patients report vibration loss at the mid-tibial or mid-ulnar area, then the complaint is hysterical, as this is a physiologic impossibility.

When patients claim complete loss of sensation in the arms or legs, the clinician should ask them to close their eyes and perform the finger to nose and heel to shin test. In true sensory deprivation a pseudoathetosis is noted in the digits, as the extremities do not appreciate their position in space. However, the hysterical patient can accurately perform the task without evidence of sensory ataxia.

I have seen several hysterical patients demonstrate complete analgesia-anesthesia to gross pressure, joint stretching and even to thermal burns. Yet, if the physician can retest the patient while he is asleep, sensation can be demonstrated by witnessing withdrawal movements from noxious stimuli. (Sleep observations are also of value in alleged motor paralysis and deafness.) This apparent dichotomy demonstrates the power and protection of the conversion symptom.

Pain

Perhaps the most common and perplexing subjective symptom confronting the clinician is the complaint of pain. This has been described in many ways with involvement of multiple body areas. Physicians are all trained to treat acute pain but when one applies these same principles to symptoms lasting more than six months (chronic), the results are disappointing. Frustration usually develops on the part of the physician due to lack of response to various therapies and ultimately these patients are labelled psychogenic. While this is not a homogeneous population several categories are observed: 1) depressed patients with severe psychiatric problems, 2) hysterics and manipulative groups of patients, 3) obscure organic dysfunction that defies standard diagnosis. All of these groups are seen in physicians' offices and also in "pain clinics." Initially it is most difficult to determine grouping of patients. In an attempt to clarify the situation, Dr. Nelson Hendler of Johns Hopkins devised a ten minute screening test to help categorize and predict outcome. This Hendler screening test (pp. 46–50) consists of a series of 15 questions that are asked of the patient and scored by the examiner. The questions that were selected had a high degree of correlation with either physical findings or surgical outcomes. Each answer has a point value. A score of 18 points or less suggests that the pain has an objective and treatable basis and organicity is to be searched for. A score of 19–31 points indicates a minimal chance of organicity and a high tendency for an exaggerated response. It is in this group that surgery and other intervention procedures should be offered sparingly and cautiously. A score greater than 32 points demonstrates depression and anxiety and suggests the need for psychiatric consultation.

Hysterics and manipulative individuals comprise a significant majority of pain populations and again several generalizations can be made of this group. Usually these patients are impeccably dressed, yet describe their agonizing pain vividly, indicating a lack of response to all therapy and an inability to sleep. They usually have a bland and detached affect ("*la belle indifference*," Fig. 1), yet describe vividly the "burning nail through the head," the "lightning-bolt onset," and the "twisting-torture-like syndrome" they are experiencing. These complaints are continuous, and are unyielding to analgesics, narcotics, nerve blocks, transcutaneous stimulation (TENS), biofeedback and acupuncture, yet they do not resemble the haggard and almost cachectic-appearing patients with thalamic syndrome or tic douloureux. The availability of unemployment insurance, disability payments, workman's compensation benefits, no-fault and other litigation aspects greatly influences how a patient handles pain, its tendency to spread to adjacent areas of the body and the rate of recovery. As noted in Table 4, different areas of the body tend to be involved more in men than in women or vice versa and in adults than in children or vice versa. Women tend to complain of pelvic discomfort more than any other body area and this is reflected in a high incidence of hysterectomy in this group. In a specific study Martin and co-workers noted a 27% incidence of hysteria prior to surgery and Cohen reported that gynecological operations were seven times more frequent in hysterics than in control subjects. They did not feel there was any excess uterine pathology in this group. The suggestion was made that when hysteria was suspected therapeutic decisions regarding hysterectomy be based only on *objective* signs and findings rather than on subjective complaints. Hendler's

TABLE 4.
Patterns of Hysterical Pain

Females—face, abdomen, vagina
Males—back, chest
Children—abdomen

Hendler 10-Minute Screening Tes for Chronic Back Pain Patients

Instructions: Each question is asked by an examiner, and the patient is given poin according to the response that he makes. The number of points to be awarded for th various responses is shown in the column at the right. At the end of the test, th examiner calculates the total number of points. The results are interpreted a explained in the **Key.**

		Points
I	**How did the pain that you now experience occur?**	
	(a) Sudden onset with accident or definable event	0
	(b) Slow, progressive onset without acute exacerbation	1
	(c) Slow, progressive onset with acute exacerbation without accident or event	2
	(d) Sudden onset without an accident or definable event	3
II	**Where do you experience the pain?**	
	(a) One site, specific, well-defined, consistent with anatomical distribution	0
	(b) More than one site, each well-defined and consistent with anatomical distribution	1
	(c) One site, inconsistent with anatomical considerations, or not well-defined	2
	(d) Vague description, more than one site, of which one is inconsistent with anatomical considerations or not well-defined or anatomically explainable	3

		Points
III	**Do you ever have trouble falling asleep at night, or are you ever awakened from sleep?** If the answer is "no," score 3 points and go to question IV. If the answer is "yes," proceed: **What keeps you from falling asleep, or what awakens you from sleep?**	
IIIA	(a) Trouble falling asleep every night due to pain	0
	(b) Trouble falling asleep due to pain more than three times a week	1
	(c) Trouble falling asleep due to pain less than three times a week	2
	(d) No trouble falling asleep due to pain	3
	(e) Trouble falling asleep which is not related to pain	4
IIIB	(a) Awakened by pain every night	0
	(b) Awakened from sleep by pain more than three times a week	1
	(c) Not awakened from sleep by pain more than twice a week	2

	Points
(d) Not awakened from sleep by pain	3
(e) Restless sleep, or early morning awakening with or without being able to return to sleep, both unrelated to pain	4

IV Does weather have any effect on your pain?

(a) The pain is always worse in both cold *and* damp weather.	0
(b) The pain is always worse with damp weather *or* with cold weather.	1
(c) The pain is occasionally worse with cold or damp weather.	2
(d) The weather has no effect on the pain.	3

V How would you describe the type of pain that you have?

(a) Burning; or sharp, shooting pain; or pins and needles; or coldness; or numbness	0
(b) Dull, aching pain, with occasional sharp, shooting pains not helped by heat; or, the patient is experiencing hyperesthesia	1
(c) Spasm-type pain, tension-type pain, or numbness over the area, relieved by massage or heat	2
(d) Nagging or bothersome pain	3
(e) Excruciating, overwhelming, or unbearable pain, relieved by massage or heat	4

	Points
VI How frequently do you have your pain?	
(a) The pain is constant	0
(b) The pain is nearly constant, occurring 50%-80% of the time	1
(c) The pain is intermittent, occurring 25%-50% of the time	2
(d) The pain is only occasionally present, occurring less than 25% of the time.	3

VII Does movement or position have any effect on the pain?

(a) The pain is unrelieved by position change or rest, and there have been previous operations for the pain.	0
(b) The pain is worsened by use, standing, or walking; and is relieved by lying down or resting the part.	1
(c) Position change and use have variable effects on the pain.	2
(d) The pain is not altered by use or position change, and there have been no previous operations for the pain.	3

VIII What medications have you used in the past month?

(a) No medications at all	0
(b) Use of non-narcotic pain relievers; non-benzodiazepine tranquilizers; or use of antidepressants	1
(c) Less than three-times-a-week use of a narcotic, hypnotic, or benzodiazepine	2
(d) Greater than four-times-a-week use of a narcotic, hypnotic, or benzodiazepine	3

	Points
IX What hobbies do you have, and can you still participate in them?	
(a) Unable to participate in hobbies that were formerly enjoyed	0
(b) Reduced number of hobbies or activities relating to a hobby	1
(c) Still able to participate in hobbies but with some discomfort	2
(d) Participate in hobbies as before	3
X How frequently did you have sex and orgasms before the pain, and how frequently do you have sex and orgasms now?	
(a^1) Sexual contact, prior to pain, three to four times a week, with no difficulty with orgasm; now sexual contact is 50% or less than previously, and coitus is interrupted by pain	0
(a^2) (For people over 45) Sexual contact twice a week, with a 50% reduction in frequency since the pain	0
(a^3) (For people over 60) Sexual contact once a week, with a 50% reduction in frequency of coitus since the onset of pain	0
(b) Pre-pain adjustment as defined above (a^1-a^3), with no difficulty with orgasm: now loss of interest in sex and/or difficulty with orgasm or erection	1
(c) No change in sexual activity now as opposed to before the onset of pain	2
(d) Unable to have sexual contact since the onset of pain, and difficulty with orgasm or erection *prior* to the pain	3
(e) No sexual contact prior to the pain, or absence of orgasm *prior to* the pain	4
XI Are you still working or doing your household chores?	
(a) Works every day at the same pre-pain job or same level of household duties	0
(b) Works every day but the job is not the same as pre-pain job, with reduced responsibility or physical activity	1
(c) Works sporadically or does reduced amount of household chores	2
(d) Not at work, or all household chores are now performed by others	3
XII What is your income now compared with before your injury or the onset of pain, and what are your sources of income?	
(a) Any one of the following scores 1. Experiencing financial difficulty with family income 50% or less than previously 2. Was retired and is still retired	0

	Points
3. Patient is still working and is not having financial difficulties.	
(b) Experiencing financial difficulty with family income only 50%-75% of the pre-pain income	1
(c) Patient unable to work, and receives some compensation so that the family income is at least 75% of the pre-pain income	2
(d) Patient unable to work and receives no compensation, but the spouse works and family income is still 75% of the pre-pain income	3
(e) Patient doesn't work, yet the income from disability or other compensation sources is 80% or more of gross pay before the pain; the spouse does not work	4
XIII Are you suing anyone, or is anyone suing you, or do you have an attorney helping you with compensation or disability payments?	
(a) No suit pending, and does not have an attorney	0
(b) Litigation is pending, but is not related to the pain.	1
(c) The patient is being sued as the result of an accident	2
(d) Litigation is pending or workmen's compensation case with a lawyer involved	3
XIV If you had three wishes for anything in the world, what would you wish for?	
(a) "Get rid of the pain" is the only wish.	0
(b) "Get rid of the pain" is one of the three wishes	1
(c) Doesn't mention getting rid of the pain, but has specific wishes usually of a personal nature such as for more money, a better relationship with spouse or children, etc.	2
(d) Does not mention pain, but offers general, non-personal wishes such as for world peace	3
XV Have you ever been depressed or thought of suicide?	
(a) Admits to depression; or has a history of depression secondary to pain and associated with crying spells and thoughts of suicide	0
(b) Admits to depression, guilt, and anger secondary to the pain	1
(c) Prior history of depression before the pain or a financial or personal loss prior to the pain; now admits to some depression	2
(d) Denies depression, crying spells, or "feeling blue"	3
(e) History of a suicide attempt prior to the onset of pain	4

POINT TOTAL

Key to Hendler Screening Test for Chronic Back Pain

A score of 18 points or less suggests that the patient is an objective pain patient and is reporting a normal response to chronic pain. One may proceed surgically if indicated, and usually finds the patient quite willing to participate in all modalities of therapy, including exercise and psychotherapy. Occasionally, a person with conversion reaction or post-traumatic neurosis will score less than 18 points; this is because subjective distress is being experienced on an unconscious level. Persons scoring 14 points or less can be considered objective pain patients with more certainty than those at the upper range (14-18) of this group.

A score of 15-20 points suggests that the patient has features of an objective pain patient as well as of an exaggerating pain patient. This implies that a person with a poor premorbid adjustment has an organic lesion that has produced the normal response to pain; however, because of the person's poor pre-pain adjustment, the chronic pain produces a more extreme response than would otherwise occur.

A score of 19-31 points suggests that the patient is an exaggerating pain patient. Surgical or other interventions may be carried out with caution. This type of patient usually has a premorbid (pre-pain) personality that may increase his likelihood of using or benefiting from the complaint of chronic pain. The patient may show improvement after treatment in a chronic pain treatment center, where the main emphasis is placed on an attitude change toward the chronic pain.

A score of 32 points or more suggests that a psychiatric consultation is needed. These patients freely admit to a great many pre-pain problems, and show considerable difficulty in coping with the chronic pain they now experience. Surgical or other interventions should not be carried out without prior approval of a psychiatric consultant. Severe depression, suicide, and psychosis are potential problems in this group of affective pain patients.

screening test would be most useful in this group and would serve to reinforce the decision not to operate and to consider other modalities of therapy. To emphasize this point further, Martin, in a one year followup, found that in general there was no reduction in complaints after surgery.

In general, acute pain is organic and has a protective function, whereas chronic pain has an uncertain etiology and psychological factors play a significant role. Perhaps the best example of this is the headache, one of the most common human afflictions. Migraine, sinus disease, MSG and concussion are well recognized causes of this distress. However, when this complaint becomes protracted and unresponsive, psychogenic aspects become apparent. This observation is continually validated by internists and general practitioners as well as by neurologists and physicians in headache clinics. Again the subjective discomfort is described in vivid terms of burning, twisting, boring, etc., and may be in any location. It does not awaken the patient from sleep and is not associated with the autonomic symptoms of nausea, vomiting or photophobia. Elements of depression are usually obvious and this may be primary or secondary. Workups including EEG, CAT and spinal fluid analysis tend to be negative. Recently, thermography has been used in an attempt to objectively discern any temperature gradients present in the involved areas. In several cases the painful areas were found to be several degrees cooler than normal and this has been interpreted as representing constricted blood vessels producing secondary ischemia. Friedman and Wood found that in migraine the entire affected side was colder by 1°C in 75% of patients, whereas in 10% the affected areas were warmer and in 15% there was no difference. On the other hand, cases of histaminic cephalgia (cluster) headaches demonstrated a unique thermographic pattern, with 67% of patients showing ipsilateral coldness. In many of these patients there was a lack of correlation between these objective temperature differences and the clinical activity of head pain. Thus the cool spots persisted, suggesting biochemical, and structural changes. I am sure that with the development of positron emission tomography (PET) scanning and nuclear magnetic resonance, further information will be generated on the underlying pathophysiology of these conditions.

Post-traumatic headaches are common and difficult problems. Litigation is always hovering in the background confusing the picture. Since thermography has been accepted in several courts throughout the USA, it has been suggested that this method will help to "aid the true sufferers and to weed out malingerers who are receiving undeserved disability payments" (*New York Times*). The following case described by Dr. Pierre Leroy illustrates this point.

Case: A 30 year old man suffered focal injury to right head and eye in 1977, and since then has complained of peri-orbital pain that has been unresponsive to various therapies. The workup, including thermography, was negative (Plate IV). He had to seek early retirement from his job because of these symptoms.

Lumbar and chest complaints tend to be more frequent in males and the statistics are rising at alarming rates as regards industrial accidents. Large numbers of compensation cases and automobile accident victims are constantly being followed by general practitioners, internists, neurologists and orthopedic surgeons. This large patient population not only has a negative economic impact on our country but also affects family relationships. The incentive to return quickly to work has been neutralized by the "real or imagined" benefits of the system. Invariably these patients receive extensive workups including electromyography, lumbar tomography and myelography, and are even treated with TENS, biofeedback and acupuncture. The results are usually disappointing and ultimately lead to the diagnosis of psychogenic back pain.

Case: A 50 year old truck driver sustained an "injury" on the job and complained of low back pain. Each time he had an office visit, histrionics were evident. There was no evidence of paravertebral spasm, restriction of straight-leg raising, atrophy or reflex asymmetry. One evening after an office examination, I saw him and his family at a sporting event. He appeared to move freely and without discomfort. To avoid embarrassing him with his family present, I telephoned him the following day and arranged an appointment. When confronted by my observation, he exclaimed that he "suddenly" felt much better after my examination and wanted to go out with his family. However, the following day he "threw his back out" and the pain was unbearable. Psychiatric consultation was recommended but refused. This type of case is essentially a prototype of cases seen frequently by physicians and leads to a great deal of personal frustration.

It should be stated at this point that often the diagnosis of psychogenic back pain is unjustified in some patients despite the fact that they have negative EMG/myelograms, etc. We must realize as physicians that these diagnostic tests are not 100% accurate and that there are several pain syndromes that are obscure and not well publicized such as myofascial pain, facet syndrome and sympathetic reflex dystrophy. In these patients the only way to establish these diagnoses is by thermography. Of 224 patients referred to the psychiatrist for evaluation of "psychogenic pain" diagnosed by orthopedic surgeons, neurologists and neurosurgeons, abnormal thermography in the affected limb (1°C or greater reduction) was found in 43 of the patients (19%). These abnormal thermograms were attributable to either reflex sympathetic dystrophy, nerve irritation or facet syndrome (Hendler). Uematsu and co-workers found a higher percentage (54%) of abnormal thermographs in chronic pain sufferers. The point to be made by these two series is that despite a negative "routine workup" an unjustified psychiatric label was applied.

Thermography is another useful test, although it has its limitations and its critics. One of its major drawbacks has been the lack of correlation of thermographic findings with clinical complaints and observations. Additionally, technical aspects, such as room temperature, can lead to error. Despite these aspects at least four states (New York, California, Wisconsin and Illinois) now accept thermographic evidence as objective proof or disproof of pain in Worker's Compensation and personal injury cases. The following two cases of Dr. LeRoy demonstrate the applications of thermography.

Case: A 62 year old female developed extensive shingles over the dorsal-lumbar region posteriorly. She experienced soreness and burning, shooting pain over a widespread area of T8-S1. A thermogram of this area confirmed the areas of relative hypothermia (arrows) over the left lattissimus dorsi muscle with differences of temperature 1–3°C (Plate V).

Case: A 24 year old female was involved in a head-on collision and suffered multiple soft tissue injuries. Numerous complaints persisted with a burning sensation on back and legs, difficulty with defecation and leg weakness. She was unresponsive to various modalities of therapy and the workup was negative. Thermography was also normal (Plate VI).

Children tend to have a high incidence of recurring abdominal pains. Sometimes the precipitating source is obvious, but at other times the conflicts are obscure. Many children ultimately reach the point of having clinical investigations with an upper GI series, an appendectomy or exploratory surgery. Recently, Barr and co-workers demonstrated lactose intolerance as a cause of repeated bouts of abdominal pain in healthy school children.

Psychodynamically speaking, pain is frequently associated with punishment and this association may be exaggerated in children who are overdisciplined; conversely, other children receive love and attention only when they sustain a painful injury or illness. Thus, later in life, they may exaggerate a minor discomfort or hallucinate a past pain in an attempt to gain security and love. Thus, pleasure and pain are intertwined.

Ethnicity has often been assumed to play a role in pain response, but in a recent study by Flannery and workers, there was no significant difference in episiotomy pain among five ethnic groups (Blacks, Italians, Jewish, Irish and Anglo-Saxon Protestants).

However, it cannot be denied that individuals exist who by nature are prone to suffer pain as determined by their personal histories and personality development. Usually, there is conflict marked by ambivalence. Typically, they manifest recurrent patterns or have polysurgery, even though organic signs are rare. The problem is due in part to their physicians' lack of awareness of hysterical pain and in part to the patients' constant, vague and diffuse symptoms. The sympathetic physician wishes to help because he mistakenly thinks that the pain is arising from a local, organic lesion. Since the patient will ultimately be evaluated by a surgeon, it is essential to maintain a high index of suspicion. A detailed history from the patient and also family members often reveals that the symptoms are almost identical with pain learned from a previous experience or observation. Some symptoms may be iatrogenically induced in the more suggestible or intelligent patients. The physician inquiring into specific symptoms allows the patient to take on a certain value that may be used at a later time. The Hendler screening test definitely has a role to play under these circumstances.

Despite the presence of numerous sensory complaints and the absence of neurological findings, one cannot exclude the presence of early serious organic disease except by repeated examinations. Multiple sclerosis, Herpes Zoster, acute intermittent porphyria

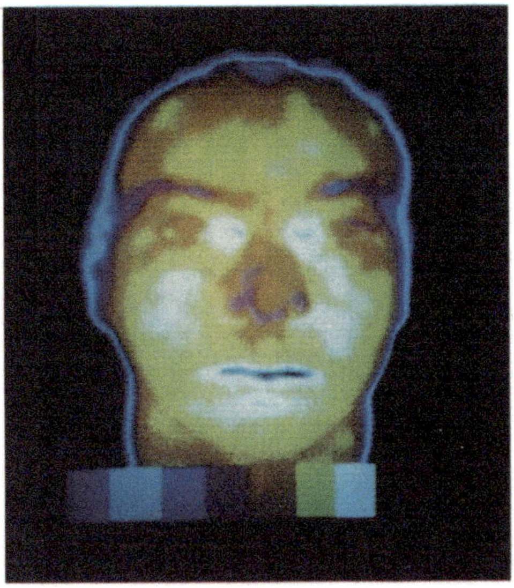

PLATE IV. Thermogram of the head of a 30 year old man complaining of peri-orbital pain.

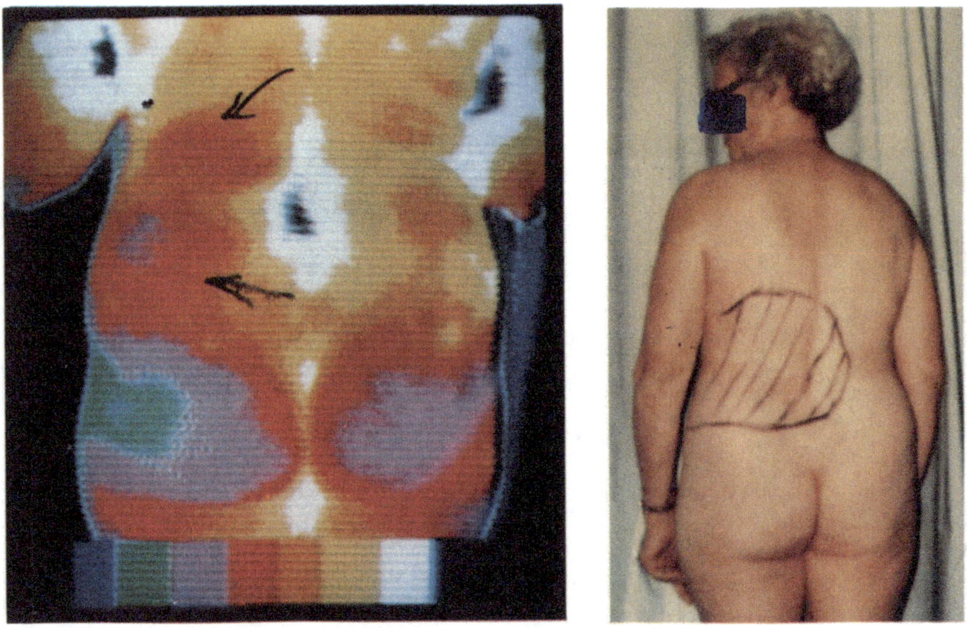

PLATE V. (left) Thermogram showing areas of relative hypothermia in a 62 year old female. (right) Area of pain drawn on the skin of this patient.

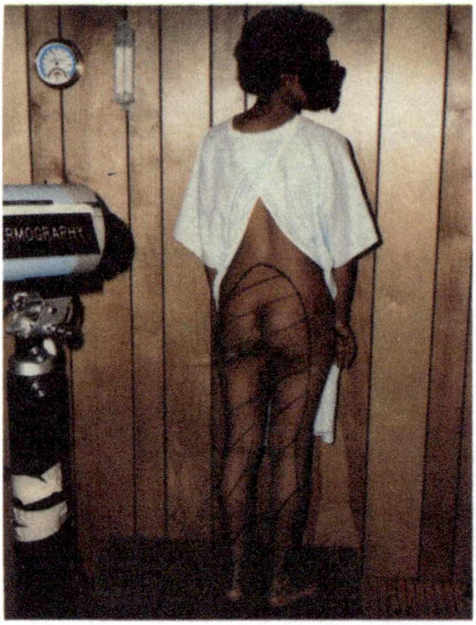

PLATE VI. (a) Twenty-four year old female complaining of a burning sensation in back and legs, difficulty with defecation and leg weakness. Thermograms (b) and (c) were normal.

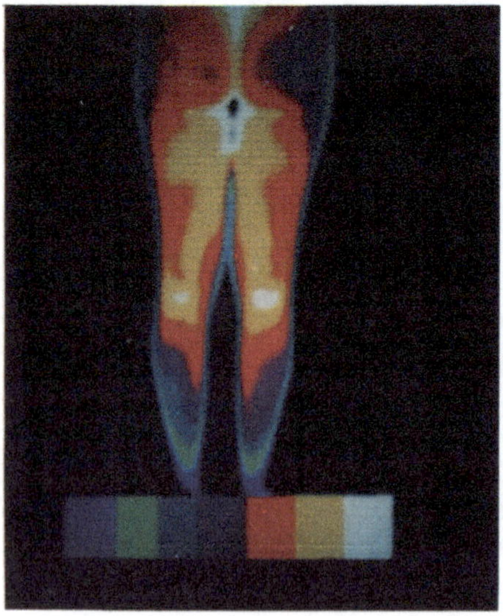

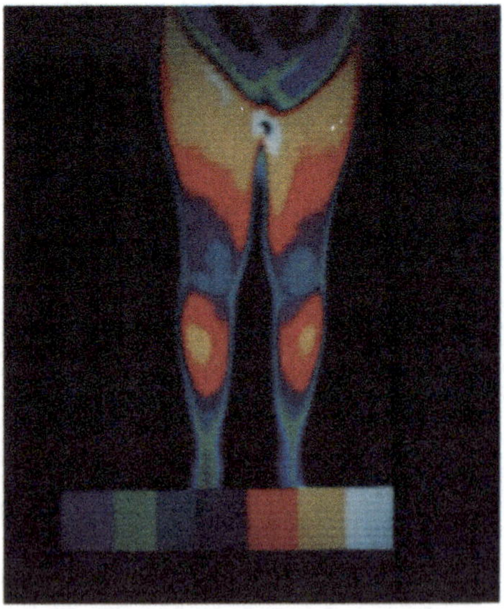

Guillain-Barre-Strohl syndrome, and causalgias may present in exactly this fashion. In cases of "whip-lash" injuries followed by excessive complaints of paresthesiae in the extremities, it is incumbent upon the physician to rule out the possibility of a small cervical canal. The same applies, but to a lesser extent, with mild lumbar injuries.

Case: A 46 year old female involved in a "whiplash" accident developed multiple complaints of neck, shoulder and arm discomfort. Occasional paresthesiae down both hands was present with weakness. Examination revealed functional sensory and motor findings. The DTR were asymmetrically depressed in the arms as compared to the legs. She was placed in cervical halter traction which intensified her symptoms. Finally, after several weeks, cervical myelography was performed revealing a markedly narrowed cervical canal. Decompressive laminectomy over several levels reversed the entire picture.

It is difficult to be precise when it comes to pain since a patient's "threshold" varies with his concentration, attention, fatigability and suggestibility. I have found that the most characteristic hysterical sensory disturbance, especially in post-traumatic cases, is diminution of cutaneous perception as well as of deep sensory stimuli over one-half of the body. It is usually on the dominant side and will also involve the head, eyes and ears even if they were not injured. In attempting to quantify and distinguish the genuineness of the complaint, the examiner can do the following:

1. vary the intensity of the stimulus and compare the sides again.
2. test dorsal and ventral areas.
3. test the corneal reflex as insensitivity cannot be feigned due to the rich plexus of nerve endings: the fifth and seventh nerves must be intact.
4. Galvanic skin responses (measures of electrical skin resistance) can be compared.
5. check for pupillary dilatation when patient is complaining of intense pain.
6. determine if TENS changes their sensitivity.

As valuable as these procedures are, they cannot by themselves be regarded as absolute in distinguishing hysteria from organicity. All too often, we as physicians are confronted with patients who have organic dysfunction, yet who, on examination, display hysterical sensory findings of which they do not complain. The significance of this is not clear, but perhaps represents the patient's subjective dismay at being ill, or perhaps is an elaboration or embellishment of illness for sympathy or demonstration of validity. In any event, the physician should be cautious in diagnosing an HCR based *only* on the sensory examination.

MOTOR DISTURBANCES

Anatomy of Motor System (Fig. 7)

The pyramidal tract fibers arise in the pre and motor areas travelling down the brain stem to decussate in the medulla. Some fibers innervating the face and bulbar areas leave at the midbrain-pontine level. After the decussation, the fibers cross and descend as the lateral cortico-spinal tract. Damage to this pathway, before the synapse, produces the characteristic upper motor neuron lesion. This is initially a flaccid paralysis which over a period of a few weeks develops degrees of spasticity. At the spinal cord level a synapse occurs on the anterior horn cell which then innervates the various muscles.

Motor Disturbances

One of the most dramatic displays in clinical medicine is the sudden onset of paralysis. When it occurs on an organic basis, for example, stroke, there is a flaccid paralysis of the arm, leg and/or face. This may be attended by other signs of sensory disturbance, depressed Deep Tendon Reflex (DTR), speech or visual alteration and Babinski response. This is an unmistakable picture. However, when it occurs on a hysterical basis, it is usually easy to detect because the examiner gets the impression that the patient is withholding strength. The paralysis, or paresis, most commonly affects the extremities as monoplegia, hemiplegia, or paraplegia. The tone is usually flaccid but may show signs of contracture from disuse. Rarely, there is a gegenhalten-like dystonia. The paralysis does not conform to the well-known patterns resulting from upper or lower motor neurone disease; rather, it follows a distribution conforming to the patient's conventional idea of the pertinent anatomy and his body image. In examination of the motor power of

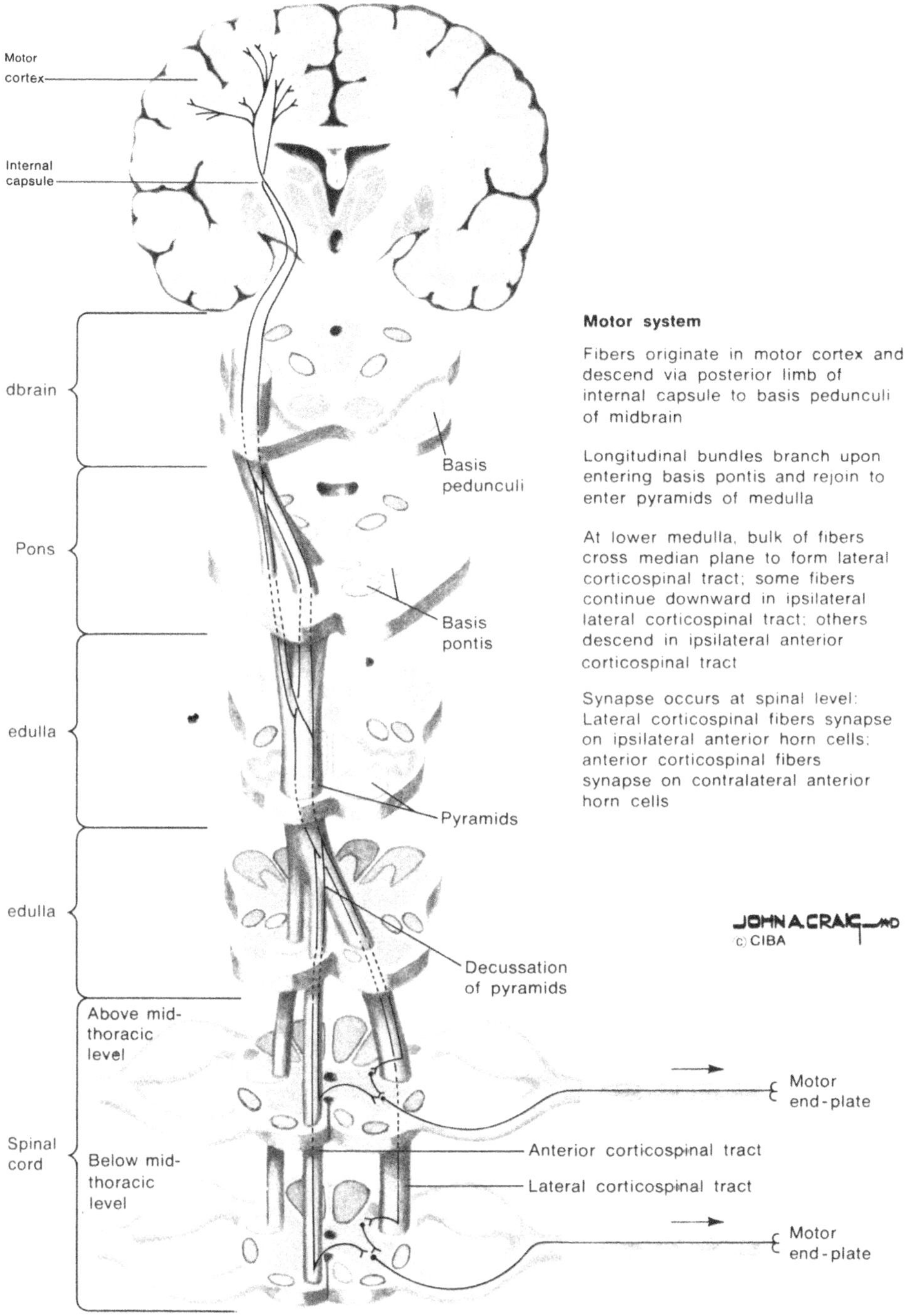

7 Descending tracts (corticospinal tracts).

Elbow flexors

1. Patient is instructed to flex arm at elbow against resistance by examiner

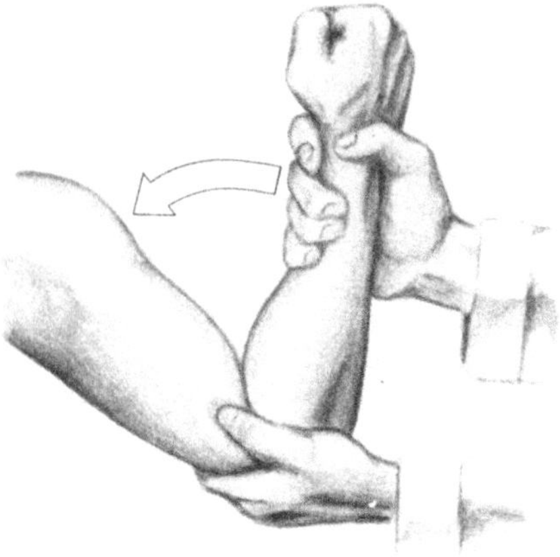

2. Examiner suddenly extends the arm, stretching flexor

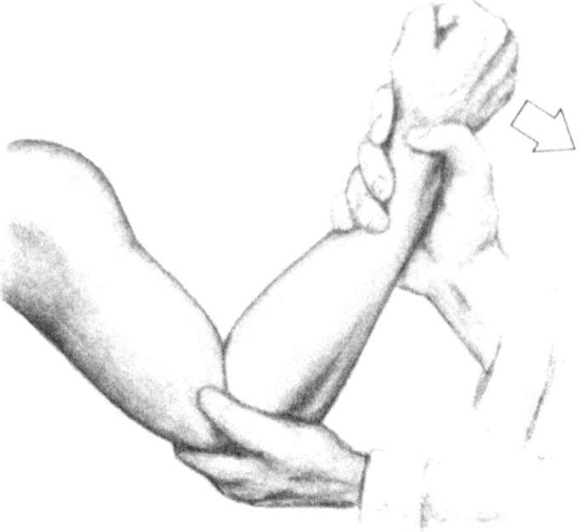

A. Response in organic paralysis

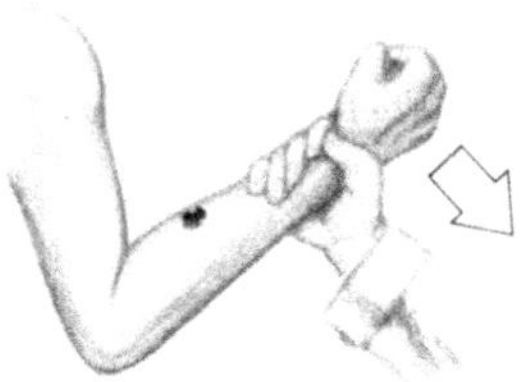

Arm is easily extended by examiner's force

B. Response in hysterical paralysis

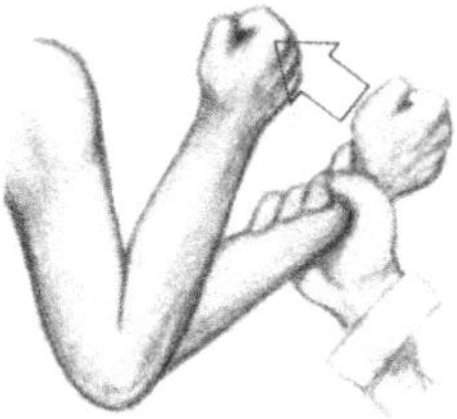

Arm extension is followed by involuntary flexion of the stretched muscle, indicating reserve strength

---

Finger flexors

1. Patient grasps examiner's fingers
2. Examiner suddenly jerks fingers back, stretching patient's flexors

A. Response in organic paralysis

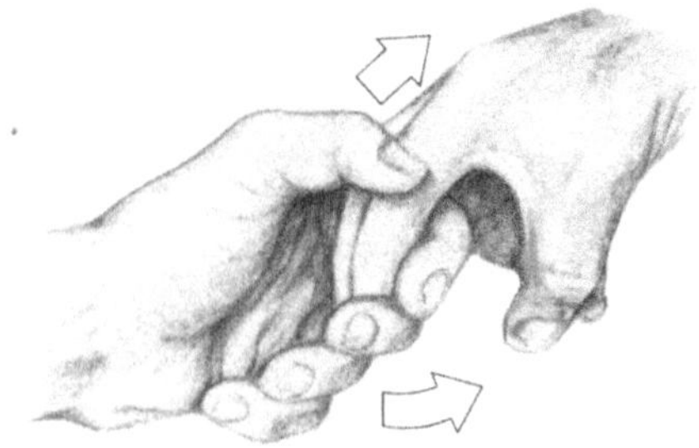

Patient's grasp is easily overpowered and examiner's fingers pull free

B. Response in hysterical paralysis

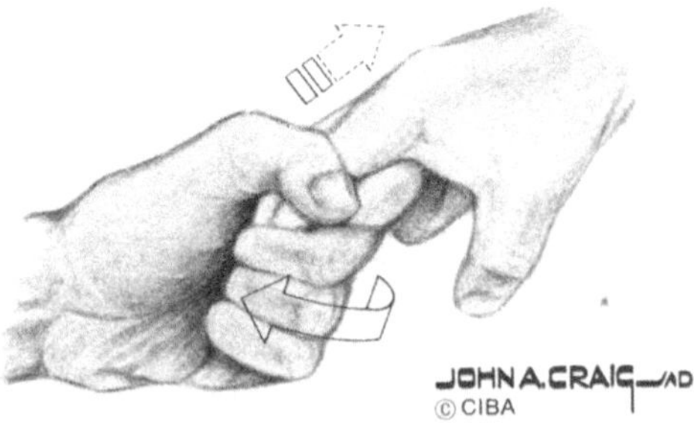

Patient involuntarily tightens grasp on examiner's fingers

8

Elbow extensors

1. Patient is instructed to extend arm at elbow against resistance by examiner

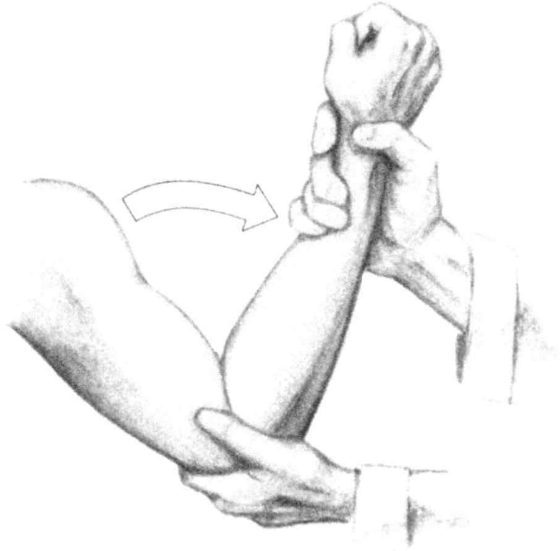

2. Examiner abruptly flexes arm backwards, stretching extensor

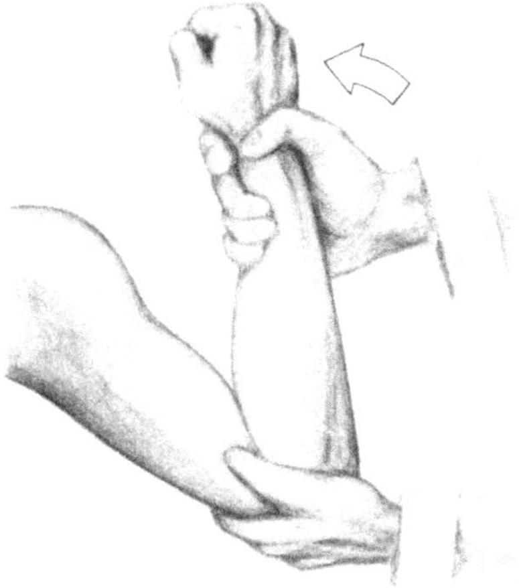

A. Response in organic paresis

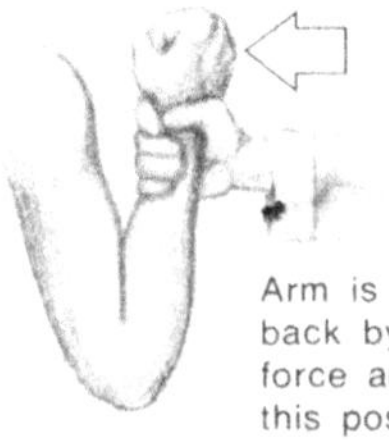

Arm is easily thrust back by examiner's force and remains in this position

B. Response in hysterical paresis

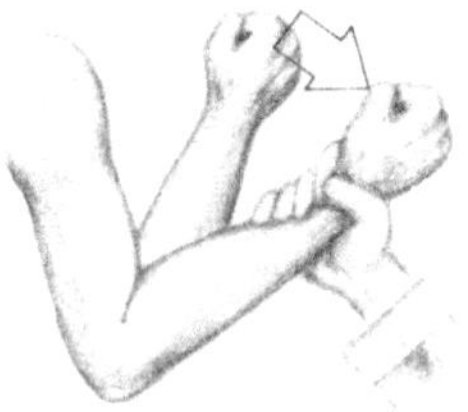

Initial passive flexion is followed by involuntary extension as muscle "unloads" reserve strength

---

Wrist extensors

Patient is instructed to make a fist; examiner watches for synergistic extension movement of wrist

A. Response in organic paresis

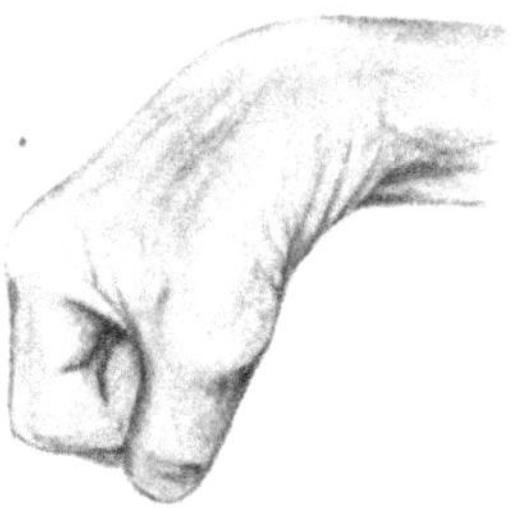

Fist is made poorly; because patient cannot extend wrist, mechanical disadvantage of flexed position impedes formation of closed fist

B. Response in hysterical paresis

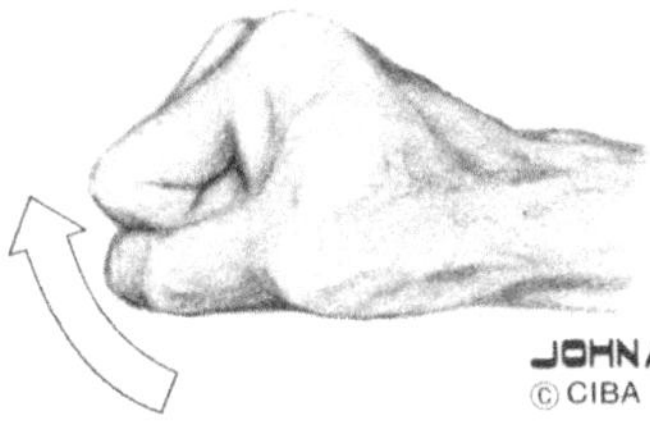

JOHN A. CRAIG AD
© CIBA

Fist is made with involuntary wrist extension to overcome mechanical disadvantage of flexed position; reserve strength is demonstrated

9 Tests for extensor weakness in upper extremity (Figures 8 and 9)

an "alleged" paresis, it should be noted that the patient makes little or no effort to contract the specific muscle. When a sudden, *unexpected* pressure is exerted on these functionally weak muscles, it results in a protective unloading of those muscles with a strong counter response (Fig. 8). This is easily demonstrated with feigned triceps muscle or hand closure weakness. Functional weakness may also be expressed as the inability to make a specific movement (Fig. 9). For example, wrist extension can be performed synergistically when making a fist, yet may not be performed voluntarily. Another clinical maneuver to determine if a flaccid limb is organically or functionally induced is to place the limb over the face and then to release it; when the flaccidity is organically induced, the limb will strike the face, but in the hysteric, it will fall safely to the side, thereby preventing injury. Since these symptoms are subconscious and self-protective, it is in the patient's self-interest not to be injured. It is a well established physiological principle that muscles work synergistically so as to allow for fine and delicate movements. Forceful movements require contraction of agonists and relaxation of antagonistic muscle groups. The patient with hysterical weakness simultaneously contracts both groups (antagonists as well as prime movers). If such a "weak" extremity is lifted off the bed and the support is suddenly released, it will be noted that the limb will hover momentarily before gently falling by gravity. Another example of the patient's false understanding of body image is when the hand is "paralyzed from the wrist down, or the forearm from the elbow down or the entire arm from the shoulder down." As is well known, the loss of function in a single joint is *never* of organic origin. The motor manifestations may be more subtle and present as excessive fatigue or weakness. This turns out to be a familiar clinical presentation and often patients have associated depression. Tremors of the extremities are another frequent occurrence and these may have bizarre aspects. They will be discussed more fully in a later section.

An objective test to confirm hysterical hand grip weakness has the patient press a dynamometer with all his strength in the "good" and "bad" hands separately. The physician then records the readings and tells the patient to simultaneously squeeze with both hands. Since it is very difficult to control both hands at the same time, the readings obtained from the "good" hand will be significantly less than on the first reading.

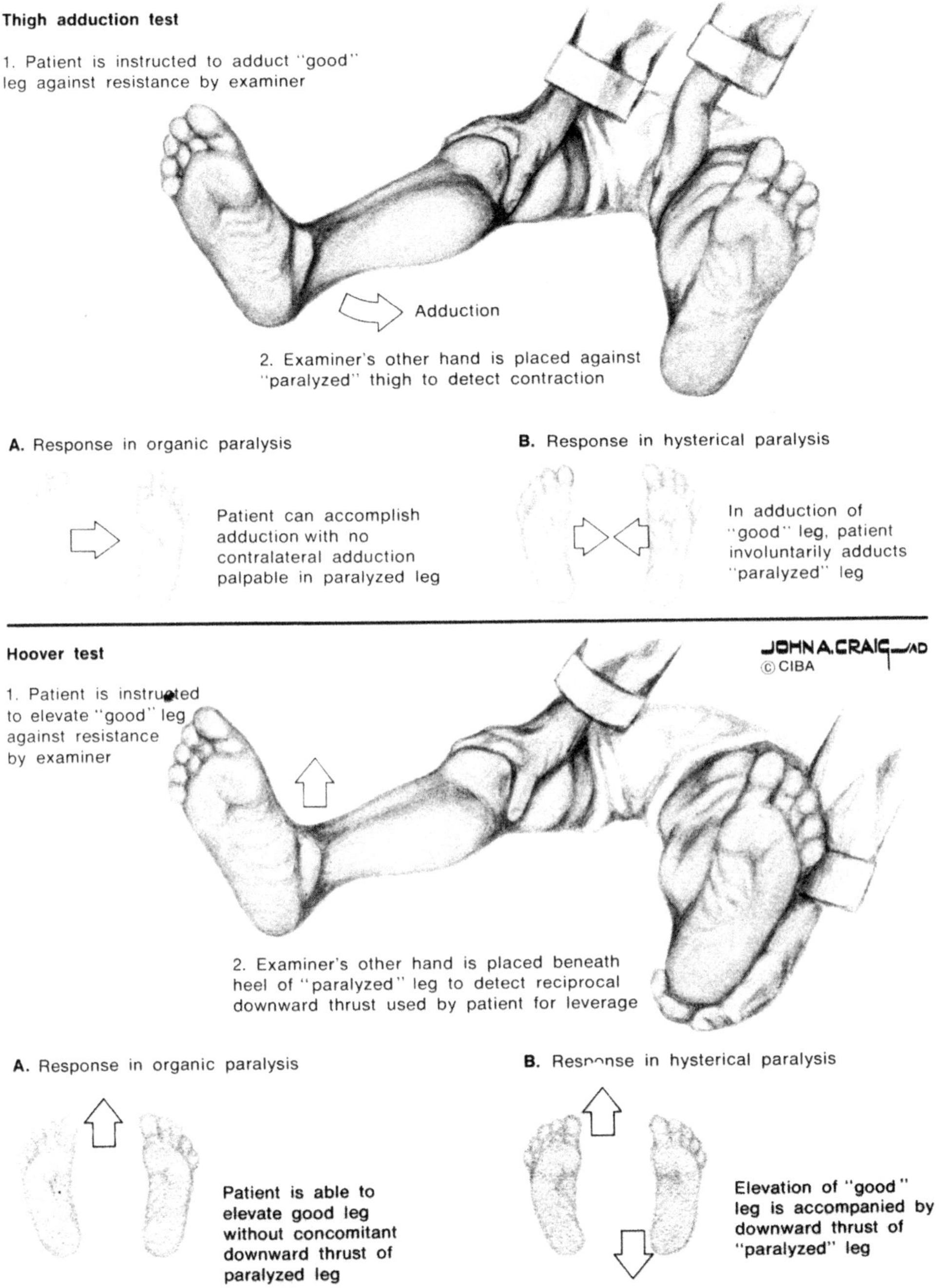

10 Tests for weakness in lower extremity.

Since well-coordinated muscle movements require simultaneous contraction and relaxation of agonistic and antagonistic muscles, this physiological fact can help the clinician diagnose hysterical leg paralysis-paresis. When the patient complains of unilateral thigh adductor weakness, the physician can feel this muscle contract as he tests the opposite (normal) thigh against resistance. Another example of this physiologic principle is incorporated in the *Hoover test* of unilateral leg paralysis. When the patient, in a supine position, attempts to lift one leg against resistance, there is normally an associated downward thrust of the other leg, which can be detected by the examiner's hand placed under the heel (Fig. 10). This associated thrust occurs in true, but not in hysterical paralysis of the opposite leg. Conversely, when the patient raises the normal leg against resistance, the hand under the heel on the affected side detects pressure in the case of hysterical paralysis, but not when it is real. A rough estimate of the pressure may be determined by placing a bathroom scale under the patient's immobile heel and measuring the number of pounds exerted. A normal adult will register between 14–18 pounds with a good effort. If there is a reduction or absence of pressure with presumed effort, this is an indication of hysterical weakness. It is very important to make multiple observations on patients with "alleged" paralysis in attempts to confirm one's suspicions. Many hysterical patients display grimacing movements, loud noises of effort, eye closure, blepharospasm, or attempted slight movement, *emphasizing their cooperation*. Sleep observations are also quite important not only for observing spontaneous movements but also the response to a noxious stimulus.
movements but also the response to a noxious stimulus.

In general, symmetrical weakness or paraplegia can be a grave sign of organicity. The diagnosis of HCR can be made if the deep reflexes and bladder function are normal and the sensory and motor signs are inconstant. However, an adept physician will rule out a parasagittal meningioma, Arnold-Chiari malformation and myelopathy. This will be a source of reassurance to the patient. The presence of normal DTRs in the setting of severe weakness is strongly suggestive of psychogenic disease, but again, the clinician should rule out myasthenia gravis, thyroid myopathy, and polymyositis which can produce similar findings (Table 5). Appropriate muscle enzyme assays (CPK, aldolase, SGOT),

TABLE 5.
Weakness with Normal Reflexes

Myasthenia gravis
Thyroid myopathy
Polymyositis
Hysteria

thyroid function and electrodiagnostic studies should clarify the picture.

Case: The author was once called into neurological consultation by a rheumatologist on the case of a 16 year old boy with severe generalized muscle weakness of arms, legs and neck muscles associated with exquisite, diffuse joint tenderness. No skin eruption was present and lab tests revealed normal sedimentation rate, ANA, CPK, EMG and muscle biopsy. An atypical (unusual) type of polymyositis was considered and patient was placed on steroids with total resolution of symptoms. As the medication was being withdrawn, the symptoms flared. Reinstitution of steroids clearly resolved the problem again. Because the treating physicians felt uncomfortable with this atypical case, a second opinion was obtained with an expert in muscle diseases and the diagnosis of HCR was made. Thus, the closer the physician is to an "organic" presentation, the more difficult to make a diagnosis. In addition, this boy had no previous emotional conflicts and was previously healthy.

Tremors with an hysterical basis are frequently seen and are produced by the simultaneous contraction of agonist and antagonist muscles. They show great variability, but often occur more frequently in the arms than the legs. Intentional movements, emotional upset or observation of extended arms, accentuate the oscillations. Proximal tremor of the shoulder or hips are almost unique to hysterics and were described extensively by Charcot. The oscillations may be gross, coarse or fine. Careful observation while eating or performing routine activity will confirm the diagnosis. Early Parkinson's disease without overt tremor, akinesia or rigidity may leave one with numerous symptoms of stiffness, fatigability or nervousness. A complete examination, however, with the findings of reduced arm swing when walking, seborrhea, greasy skin and tendency to stare, may suggest the early diagnosis of basal ganglionic disease.

Torticollis and kyphosis are usually organic syndromes but may also be hysterical in origin. I recently examined a woman who kept her neck in a wry position for several years. She was seen by numerous physicians and received many medications without relief. A detailed history indicated that she was almost strangled at an early age by a young man and this thought resurfaced just prior to the onset of this symptom. As the patient was encouraged to talk about her feelings and fright her neck was noted to assume a more normal posture.

GAIT DISORDERS

Inability to walk due to leg weakness is not an infrequent occurrence. Bizarre gait patterns are seen which are individualized to meet the patient's needs and which conform to the type of motor disability which the patient imagines he has. For example, some patients can only walk with assistance and, if left alone, seek the support of adjacent furniture or the examiner. Other patients attempt to walk and always fall to the side of support. Some walk with a zigzag gait, lurching from one source of support to another without injuring themselves and rarely falling. Actually, this type of hysterical gait requires complex muscle coordination to prevent falling. After observing their behavior, it is a good idea to place these patients in the middle of the room and continually reverse their positions to determine if a specific pattern emerges. Patients with organic ataxia fall in a random manner. It is also a good idea for the physician to check the soles and heels of both shoes to determine if they are equally worn down. Occasionally, malingerers will put on a demonstration only in the presence of doctors. Some patients clearly refuse to place weight on their legs and on standing, promptly fall to the floor claiming weakness. If the strength of the legs is tested while the patient is in bed and found to be normal, then the diagnosis of astasia-abasia is confirmed (Fig. 11). From an organic standpoint the clinician must make sure there is no disease of the anterior lobe of the cerebellum or the parasagittal area. A cervical spinal cord lesion must also be ruled out. Astasia-abasia is quite rare but usually manifests itself in males under acute stress. Hammer described two cadets subjected to extreme psychological and physiological stress who felt they could not live up to the masculine image of West Point. In a supportive atmosphere these symptoms disappeared.

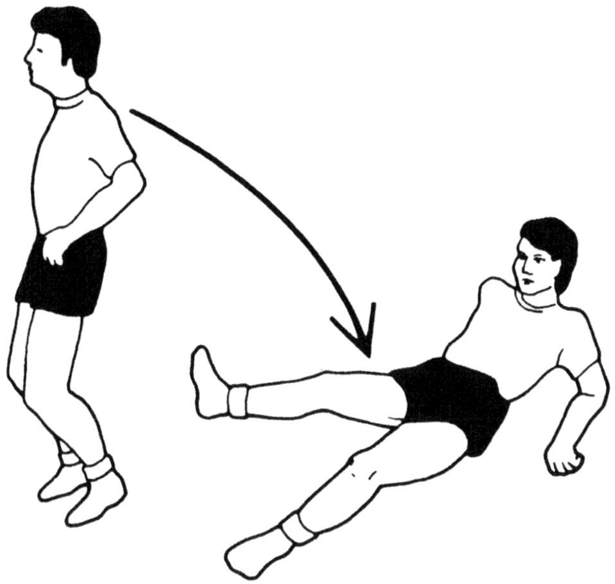

11 Astasia-abasia: inability to walk despite excellent strength in legs.

A common hysterical gait pattern is the dragging of one leg inertly. The foot is rotated outward and there is contact on the medial side of the foot with the floor. There are no circumduction movements or Babinski sign as may be observed in pyramidal tract dysfunction.

Case: A seventeen year old boy who started heavy alcohol consumption, to the point of being an alcoholic, complained of constant pain in the right lower quadrant, but medical workups were unrevealing. Because of persistence of complaints, an exploratory abdominal operation was performed, with removal of the appendix. No local pathology was found. The symptoms persisted after surgery. The patient became depressed and was admitted to a local psychiatric hospital. Neurological consultation was requested, to delineate the strange pain syndrome and the altered gait. Classic leg dragging was noted with associated functional alterations in motor strength and sensory perception. Family history revealed an overpowering mother and it was believed that he symbolically attempted to separate from his intolerable home situation via these symptoms. There was no evidence of acute intermittent porpyria.

Case: Recently a nineteen year old graduating dental hygienist developed progressive leg weakness and paralysis while taking final examinations. Because she had had a mild respiratory infection a few days before, she was admitted to rule out possible GBS syndrome. Examination revealed a positive Hoover test, hyperactive DTRs, *la belle indifference* and moderate suggestability (LP & EMG were normal). Suggestion allowed her to walk. She was informed that her emotional state overwhelmed her and symbolically prevented her from making the most important decision in her life — to leave home and pursue a new career.

The presentation of a robot gait with stiff extended legs is rarely seen. However, the clinician must be aware of a rare condition known as the *Stiff-man syndrome* in which the patient has episodic muscle aches and tightening of the axial muscles. Over time the tightness becomes constant, generalized and ultimately restrains voluntary movements. Associated with the persistent muscle rigidity are paroxyms of muscle spasms lasting several minutes. The sensory and reflex examinations are normal but the EMG is confirmatory with a pattern of constant firing even when the patient is attempting to relax. There is no evidence of myotonia. Diazepam and Baclofen have been useful. (Miller and Korsvik)

Disorders of Coordination

Occasionally patients demonstrate altered coordination in the upper extremities. This can be demonstrated to be hysterical by the finger-to-nose test (Fig. 12). When the disorder is functional, instead of accurately reaching the nose, the finger or hand takes a deviant but accurate course to the nose, or else the finger will consistently reach another site (eye, ear).

Writer's cramp has been considered by some neurologists to be functional in that these patients are unable to sign their name, yet they demonstrate agility and dexterity using the same muscles when playing a piano or shuffling cards. Others feel this is a manifestation of segmental dystonia and can be an isolated finding or part of the constellation of dystonia musculorums deformans.

Physicians unfamiliar with certain movement disorders, especially dystonia, are often misdiagnosing these patients as HCR. Lesser and Fahn reviewed 84 patients with idiopathic torsion dystonia and found 37 cases misdiagnosed as HCR. The

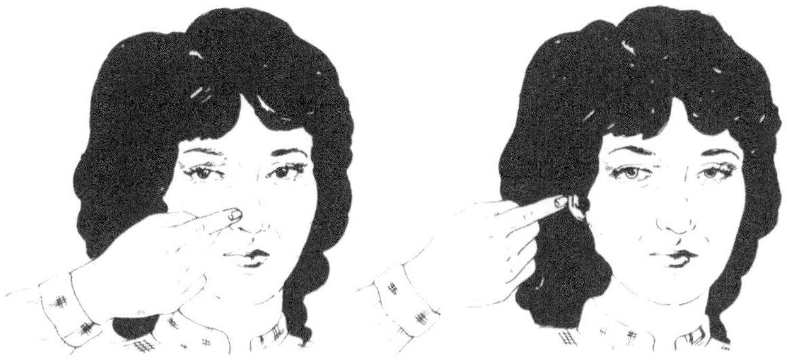

12 Finger to nose test. Note the excellent coordination to a "wrong" body part.

reasons are obvious when one encounters any of the following: tonic twisting of the neck (torticollis) that disappears with touching the chin; ability to walk backwards but not forwards; able to run but not walk; ability to sing but not talk; spasms of the eyelids while reading but absent while watching television; disappearance of the spasms while asleep; intensification of symptoms when anxious; absence of family history. (Lesser and Fahn)

Other types of bizarre movement disorders have also been reported which appear to have an organic basis in that they respond to L-dopa or anticonvulsants. These paroxysmal, recurrent, brief and stereotyped attacks of posturing and writhing have been called Paroxysmal Kinesiogenic Choreathetosis and these patients characteristically have intact consciousness, amnesia is not present and there is a normal neurological and EEG exam. (Waller, D.A.)

Case: A 27 year old homosexual became intoxicated with angel dust and was brought to the hospital. Shortly thereafter, his roommate was mugged and murdered. When the patient recovered he developed bizarre head jerking. He was able to acknowledge his guilt about leaving his lover, and, with supportive care, was able to function normally except when agitated.

Case: A 46 year old female presented with bizarre torticollis, choking sounds, facial contortions and violent neck jerking into flexion and extension. The attacks lasted five minutes without loss of consciousness or involvement of other body parts. An EEG was normal during one such attack (Fig. 26). There was no post-ictal sleepiness. A review of her past history revealed that her first husband beat her and nearly choked her at age 28. He also stabbed her behind the left ear. Shortly thereafter he was murdered in a knife fight and she developed torticollis and similar symptoms. She received psychotherapy and after a few years, these symptoms subsided. She remarried and did well except for sporadic symptoms.

Other patients manifest incoordination of their upper extremities but when observed can adeptly tie their shoes, dress and undress without tremor, chorea, myoclonus or athetosis. Some claim ataxia in one or two injured digits, yet perform flawlessly with the other fingers. The physician must always consider a functional basis for complaints when a patient's "ataxic movements" are as severe with eyes open as when they are shut. Usually the visual cues allow for better performance.

The Romberg test is essentially a measure of sensory input and health rather than a test of coordination. Many hysterical patients fall as soon as their eyes are shut, without wavering or blepharospasm, and usually backward. A patient with true ataxia will attempt to prevent a fall and many associative movements will be present. Several neurologists employ a simple distraction for the patient with functional Romberg by asking them to quickly perform other maneuvers, such as touching a body part and crossing the midline. By using these rapid commands the patient's subconscious becomes distracted and forgets to sway and fall.

CRANIAL NERVE DISTURBANCES

Hysterical loss of cranial nerve functions occurs frequently in clinical practice and merits the scrupulous attention of the physician. There are numerous manifestations that can confuse the practitioner and helpful diagnostic hints will be described.

Smell

Anosmia is well known after head injury with severance of olfactory fibers at the level of the cribriform plate. The most frequent trauma site is the occipital region followed by the facial and frontal regions. It is also frequently seen in chronic smokers and occurs with olfactory groove meningiomas. However, it is rarely a manifestation of functional disease. Whenever patients complain of this, it is usually unilateral and on the side of the hysterical motor or sensory paralysis. Organic lesions rarely cause unilateral loss of smell due to the extensive crossing of fibers, as well as overflow with vapors and solutions. The distinction from organic causes can be made with the use of spirits of ammonia (Fig. 13). The hysterical patient misinterprets the irritative odor as purely an olfactory stimulus, whereas it is in reality a trigeminal nerve irritant. Thus, the hysteric denies the stimulus whereas the true anosmic patient can identify it. The physician should also

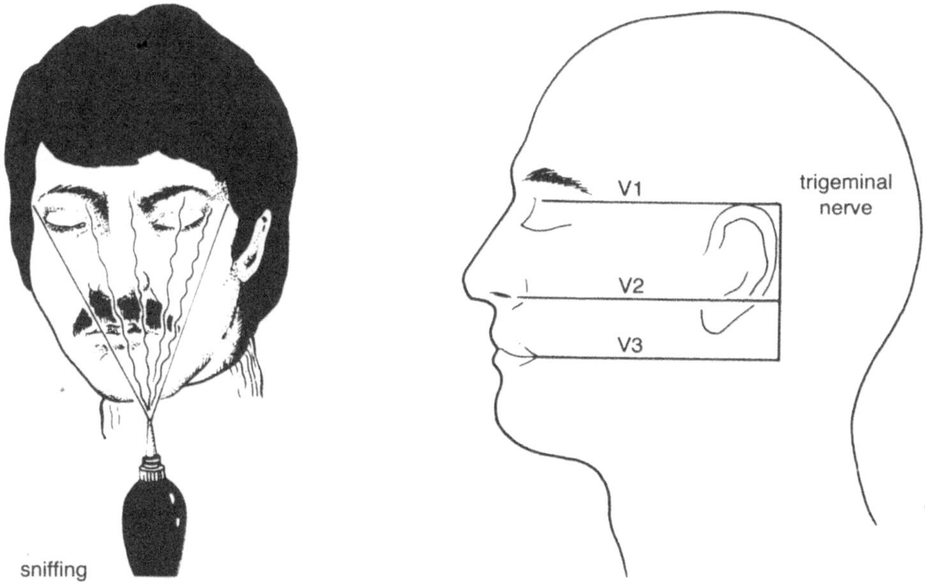

13 Olfactory test: a trigeminal nerve irritant using spirits of ammonia.

observe the patient during this maneuver to determine if there is reflex narrowing of the nostrils with a facial expression of irritation and disgust. Hysterics rarely complain of hyperosmia or paraosmia or uncinate smells. These complaints are usually perversions of the normal sensation and are usually organic reflections of temporal lobe dysfunction. This symptom can also be frequently noted in depression, local disease and Addison's Disease.

Taste

Impairment of taste (hypoageusia) or loss (ageusia) occurs with several organic syndromes including diabetes mellitus, local infection, zinc deficiency and chronic renal failure.

Taste receptors are essentially chemoreceptors that have the ability to distinguish flavors from substances dissolved in the surrounding oral fluids. The taste buds are the end organ located in the tongue papillae, mucosa of the epiglottis, soft palate and pharynx. The sensory nerve fibers on the anterior two-thirds of the tongue travel in the chorda tympanic branch of the facial nerve, whereas the posterior one-third of the tongue is innervated via the glossopharyngeal nerve. Vagal nerve branches supply the other areas of the pharynx and epiglottis.

There are four basic taste modalities and each has a predilection for different areas of the tongue (Fig. 14).

1. Sweet — at the tip
2. Sour — along the edges
3. Bitter — posterior portion of tongue
4. Salty — on the dorsum anteriorily

Identification of this sensation can be performed using standard substances, i.e., sugar for sweet; saline for salt taste, weak hydrochloric acid for sour and urea for bitter. The clinician can perform the three drop technique whereby the test solution is placed in one area and two controls of distilled water are placed nearby. If the patient recognizes the sensation, then taste appears intact. One can quantify this by increasing the concentrations of the test solutions.

It should be noted that the sense of smell is closely associated with taste sensation. If a patient with hysterical anosmia states that he is unable to smell, yet can distinguish various taste sensations, i.e., sour, bitter, salty, sweet, then his symptoms are functional. Taste alterations can also be functional and the examiner can detect

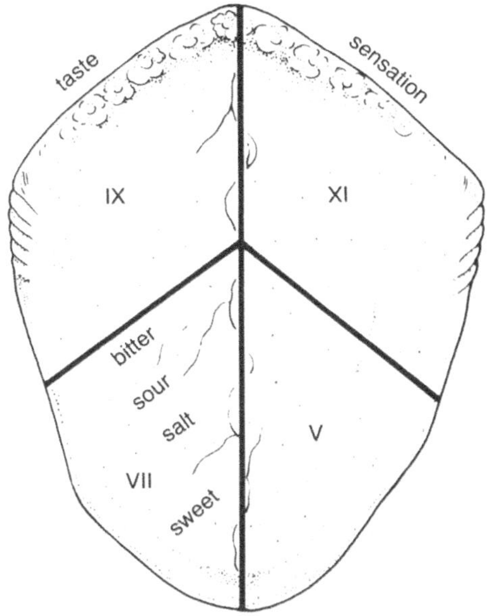

14 Functional anatomy of the tongue.

this with serial three drop technique testing. A knowledge that acids are better appreciated on the anterior portion of the tongue, whereas bitter taste is more sensitive posteriorily on the tongue and soft palate, is most helpful in coming to this conclusion.

It should be noted that the gradual development of anosmia should prompt the physician to ask specific questions regarding uncinate hallucinations, personality changes, *dejà vu* and altered levels of consciousness, and should lead to investigation of the anterior fossa to rule out a meningioma. A CAT scan would be the most appropriate screening test to determine if organic factors are present.

Visual Disturbance

Visual difficulties are by far the most common complaint and vary from total blindness to blurred vision. The range of hysterical symptoms is extensive and includes blurred vision, photophobia, diplopia, night blindness, intermittent visual failure with amnesia, altered day vision, unilateral loss of visual acuity and deficient depth perception. Air cadets have been noted to have a significant number of visual complaints when stressed, and the symptoms displayed by each patient were closely related to the stress of his performance duties.

Many patients describe a concentric narrowing of their peripheral visual fields, so that they are left only with tunnel or "gun barrel" vision. If the examiner measuring the resulting fields of vision, doubles or triples the testing distances and finds exactly the same visual field, then the patient is exhibiting hysterical visual loss because the spreading properties of light should increase the field (Fig. 15). Repeat testing may demonstrate progressively smaller and smaller fields producing a characteristic helicoid tracing. A further amplication of this maneuver is to test the visual fields in good light and then after a prolonged stay in a dark room. If there is a wider visual field after the latter, then the finding is hysterical. Likewise, if the fields are tested with a blue and red light and if the smaller field is smaller, then this finding should suggest to the clinician that the complaint is hysterical. It should be noted that chronic papilledema, retinitis pigmentosa and chronic glaucoma are some of the major organic conditions that can produce a restricted peripheral field. Obviously, a detailed medical history and detailed physical examination will indicate whether these are present.

Homonomous hemianopsia is seen only with vascular and structural lesions involving the retrogeniculate fibers and the occipital lobe; this finding is almost never due to hysteria.

Sudden unilateral blindness, with or without orbital pain, is indeed frightening and may represent optic neuritis. This condition is often confused with hysteria since the funduscopic examination is normal in both conditions. The major diagnostic criterion, however, is the pupillary response to light. Organic blindness produces a loss of the direct light reflex with retention of the consensual reflex; in psychogenic blindness however, the direct and consensual responses are retained. Another important pupillary abnormality that may be present is the Marcus-Gunn springing pupillary sign. In this test, the patient is requested to fixate on an object in the distance. There is a to-and-fro movement of bright light on the pupils within a darkened room. The light is then maintained upon one pupil and the ability to maintain constriction is noted. The test is repeated on the other pupil. With

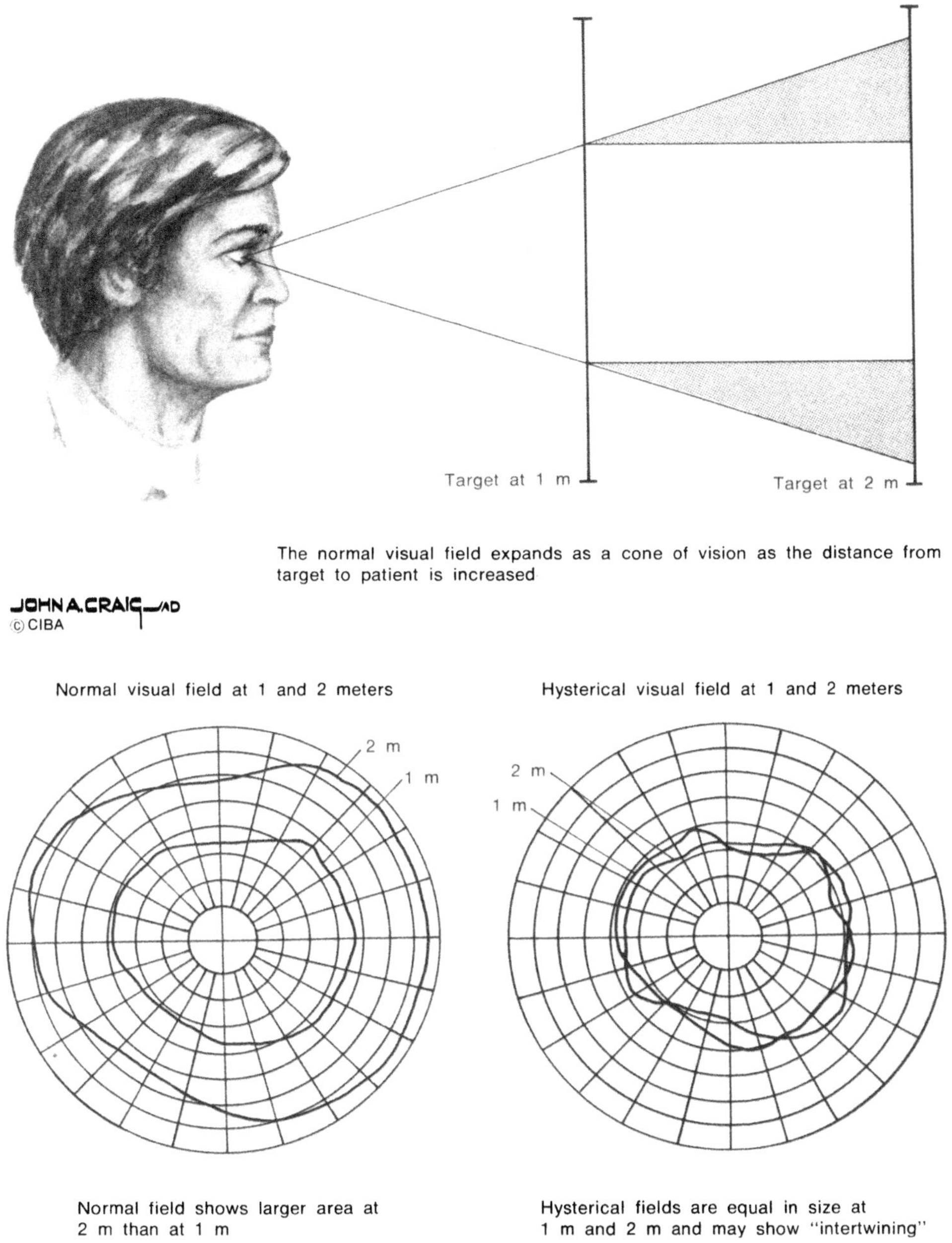

15 Visual fields.

a unilateral optic nerve lesion, the pupil is unable to maintain constriction and promptly dilates (springs). This is not present in hysterical conversion reactions. It is important to make the diagnosis of optic neuritis, as steroid treatment is usually beneficial in quickly restoring vision. The patients must also be followed up closely, as a significant percentage (30–50%) will develop multiple sclerosis.

The presence of an enlarged blind spot or central scotoma will also help establish the organic nature of the complaints. Other organic ocular lesions that must be ruled out are central retinal artery occlusion, retinal vein occlusion and amaurosis fugax.

Pupillary reactions, however, may be unreliable in patients complaining of blindness. The major source of error is those patients who have cortical blindness. In this condition, there is bilateral occipital lobe infarction or damage producing bilateral blindness but normal pupillary responses. Occlusion of the posterior cerebral arteries and carbon monoxide poisoning are two of the leading causes for this syndrome. A variation of cortical blindness is the so-called Anton syndrome whereby the patient denies that he is blind. He is often observed to stumble over objects in walking and handles objects like a blind individual. Inconsistency in the recognition of objects is the rule. Optokinetic nystagmus is absent. It is not unusual for these patients to deny, confabulate or be indifferent to the blindness. This agnosia is secondary to extension of the damage from the primary visual cortex (Brodmann's area 17) to the adjacent visual association areas (18 and 19). If one inquires about the person's background, it becomes obvious that these individuals regard ill health as a sign of weakness or imperfection and symbolically are unwilling to admit any loss of bodily functions. Recently, Cusamano and co-workers described the scintigraphic appearance of such a case.

Detection of simulated blindness is not always easy and it is important for the physician to observe patients without their knowledge. The malingerer will clearly avoid objects in his path and usually wears dark glasses.

Pupillary responses are important and can quickly localize an organic lesion (Fig. 16). Some of the more common neurological pupillary signs are represented in this diagram. In a truly blind eye, the pupil is dilated and unreactive. If a small amount of vision is preserved, then the pupil will react to light feebly. Consequently, the physician must be suspicious of a patient with

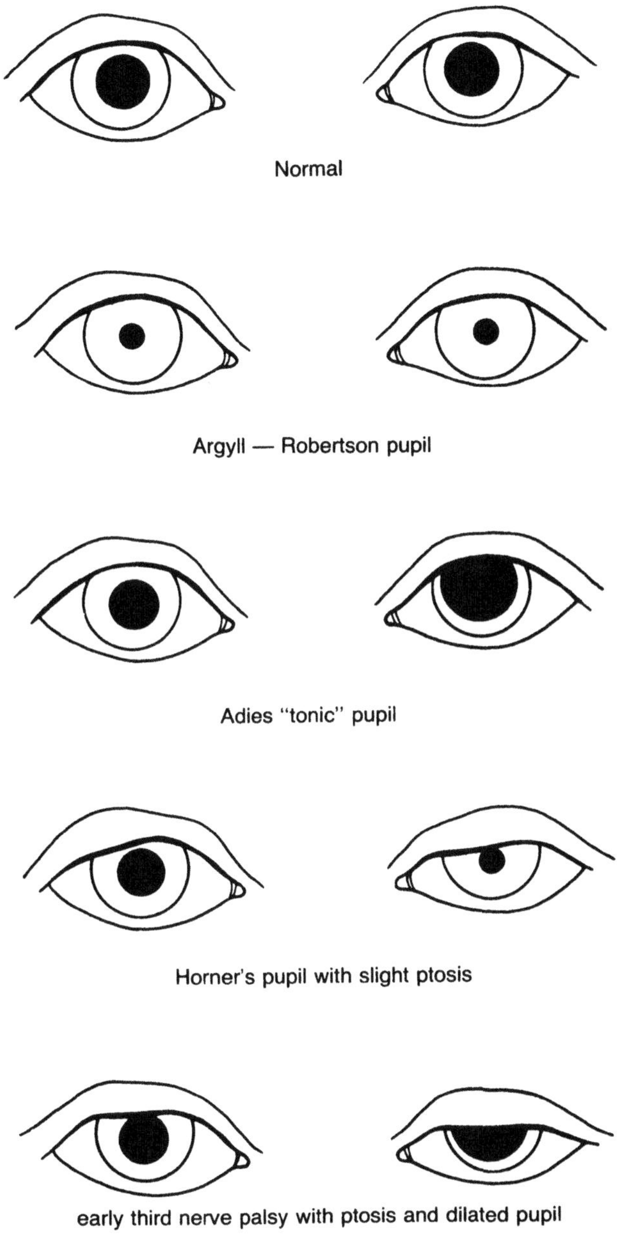

16 Common pupillary reactions.

alleged blindness with a persistently strong pupillary light reaction.

Often, malingerers will instill mydriatics into their eyes; thus, their pupils are fixed and dilated. Observations of the conjunctivae will reveal congestion and inflammation. In addition, if the patient is placed in a dark room, the normal sympathetic response would be dilatation of the pupil and if this is absent, one should suspect the presence of a cycloplegic drug.

The red glass test (Fig. 17) for unilateral blindness can also quickly indicate if the symptoms are organic or hysterical in origin. The examiner places a red glass over the "normal" eye and asks the patient to read a line of alternating black and red letters (A P E O T F—underscore indicates use of red letter). Since the red letters are invisible when looking through a red glass, the patient with hysterical blindness will read "A, P, E, O, T, F," whereas the patient with one organically blind and one normal eye will read "A, E, T."

Another useful test when confronted with a bewildering case of blindness is to apply a highly refractive magnifying glass or prism over the eye. By placing a convex lens of five diopters over the normal eye thereby making it myopic, the patient cannot read print far away. The patient is first asked to read aloud with both eyes at a short distance and then the print is gradually withdrawn farther than eight inches. If the patient continues reading, he is obviously seeing with the "allegedly defective eye." This same principle is also employed with the use of a four degree prism. The patient, believing that the lens will correct his vision, will satisfactorily identify numbers and objects at a distance. Since these prisms distort and reduce the visual acuity, the patient's vision should deteriorate, but in hysterical conversions, their actual true vision will prevail.

Some ophthalmologists place a weak concave glass (−25 diopters) before the "allegedly blind eye" and a strong plus glass (+16 diopters) before the normal eye and have the patient read. If he can see the distant type, then vision is intact. There are numerous other tests that can be employed to detect hysterical blindness, but they are complicated and require special equipment. Thus, if one suspects the symptoms to be hysterical, then an appropriate ophthalmological consultation is warranted and a definitive statement can be made by the specialist.

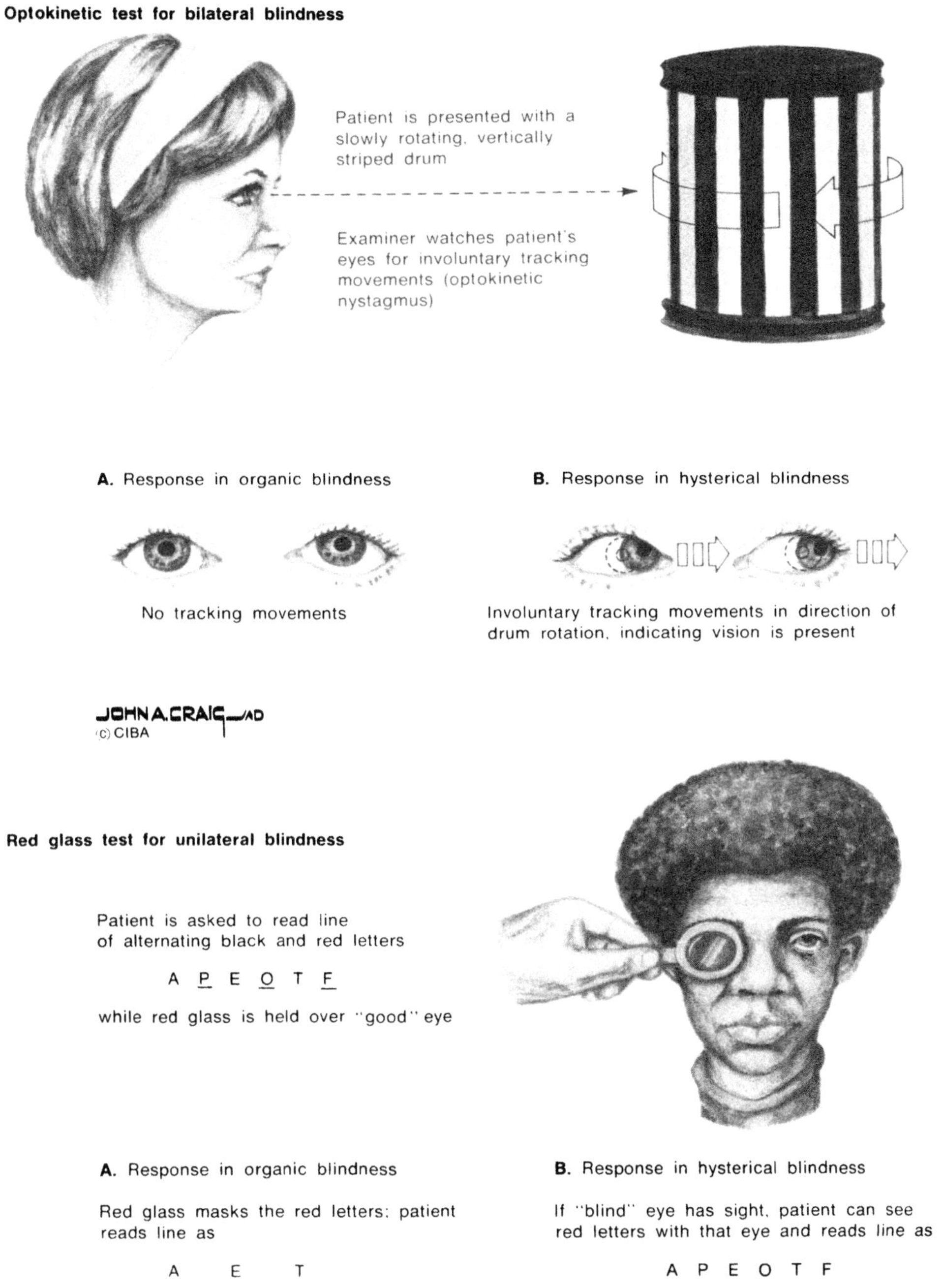

17 Tests for loss of vision.

An alleged inability to read any but the large type letters of the Snellen chart can be unmasked by knowledge of the laws of reflection. The patient is placed 20 feet from a mirror in front of a Snellen chart. After he has read the last line, he is moved 10 feet closer to the mirror and another Snellen chart with letters of the same size but printed backwards is presented and he is asked to read the letters seen in the mirror. Being half the distance from the mirror, he may read twice the number of lines he saw at the 20 foot mark, since he is ignorant of the laws of reflection.

Bilateral blindness can also be distinguished by the presence of optokinetic nystagmus to a rotating drum (Fig. 17) and response to photic stimulation on the electroencephalogram (Fig. 18). I find the response to threat to be unreliable as the movements of the examiner's hands may put pressure on the globe or eyelashes.

The study of conversion reactions in 56 male student aviators by Mucha and Reinhardt is informative. Seventy-three percent developed visual symptoms at a time when their anxiety level was extremely high due to the threat of loss of life. All were college graduates and were reared in an achievement oriented environment. They could not admit failure. Thus, when faced with an intolerable situation, the rigid superego, rather than admitting failure, converted into symptoms. In the aviation environment, visual problems prevailed, whereas in a similar study in the Army, the legs assumed a more dominant role. These studies again emphasized that both sexes can develop hysterical conversion reaction and that education attainment is not a factor.

Case: A nineteen year old college female had sudden onset of eye pain followed by blurred vision and reduced visual acuity. She was examined by her family doctor who found her eyes to be normal. Because she was in the midst of school examinations, the doctor told her it was due to her "nerves." Within two days, she developed only finger perception in the involved eye. She went to an ophthalmologist who made a diagnosis of optic neuritis and found a Marcus-Gunn pupillary sign to be present. High doses of steroids were started and within four weeks, her vision returned to normal. Six months later, she developed hemianesthesia and clumsiness. Neurological consultation confirmed the presence of multiple sclerosis.

Diplopia is a common complaint and is usually monocular. This must be considered hysterical in origin if a dislocated lens or

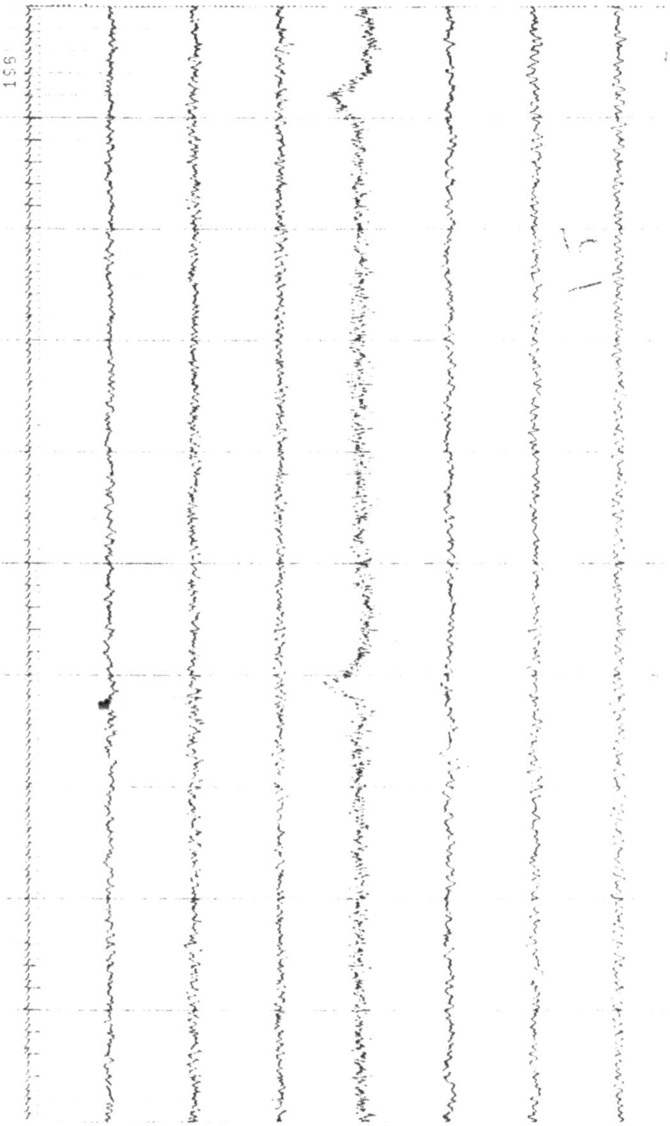

18 This demonstrates increased frequencies (harmonics) in the occipital regions in response to phonic stimulation (15 cps).

other local ocular disease can be ruled out. Binocular diplopia is usually not hysterical and most cases in young adults turn out to be multiple sclerosis. This most often arises as a result of an internuclear ophthalmoplegia from a plaque in the medial longitudinal fasciculus (MLF). The red glass test can quickly identify the specific muscle imbalance, because the involved muscle projects a false image peripheral to the true image. In genuine diplopia, the covering of either eye will allow for clear vision; however, the diplopia or triple vision will persist in the affected eye if the other eye is covered.

True paralysis of contralateral gaze is never hysterical in origin. The complaints of blepharospasm, photophobia and convergence spasm, however, are quite common in hysterical patients.

Case: Convergence spasm was so prominent in a sixteen year old girl that an inexperienced physician thought she had a brain tumor with "bilateral sixth nerve palsy." He planned a major workup until it was demonstrated that the symptoms were hysterical. The demonstration of miosis on attempted lateral gaze is a good clinical sign of spasm of the near reflex. Troost and Troost recently described the clinical maneuvers employed in diagnosing a fifty-two year old steel worker with this deficit. Meloff and co-workers described a conversion sixth nerve palsy in a child, again emphasizing the importance of a careful history and physical exam so as to avoid unnecessary testing. In their case, the obvious secondary gains were described.

Unilateral ptosis may be seen as a conversion reaction and can be easily detected by the clinician by requesting the patient to look up at the ceiling. When the patient performs this task, there is an upward contracting motion of the orbicularis oculi muscles with the contraction of the frontalis muscle. Hysterical ptosis is usually a bilateral phenomenon. Hart described a case of hysterical blepharospasm with bilateral ptosis in a woman having an extramarital affair. Hart found that the patient was "shutting her eyes" to reality, and her symptoms reversed when her repressed feelings became conscious. Krueger recently described the dynamic psychopathology in a woman with unilateral ptosis as a conversion reaction. Her symptom choice was determined by her concept of physical illness and symbolic needs. It is obvious that when the physician is confronted by a patient with bilateral ptosis, myasthenia gravis and thyroid disease must be ruled out.

Some patients have reported micropsia (objects appear unusually small), macropsia (objects seem unusually large and may be terrifying). Thus, a wide range of visual alterations can be experienced and it is up to the physician to rule out organic involvement and to determine whether the complaints are hysterical in origin.

Hysterical Deafness

Hysterical deafness is a rare symptom that can be seen at any age but tends to be more common in wartime. It may be partial, total, unilateral or bilateral. This was demonstrated in the study by Mucha and Reinhardt when 14% of the aviators developed hysterical auditory symptoms in response to a presumed threat to their lives. Hysterical deafness is most commonly unilateral.

When deafness occurs in childhood, it may have selective elements, i.e., it only occurs with certain people or under certain circumstances. The bedside examination is usually unsatisfactory and formal audiometric testing is often required. However, there are several bedside techniques and clinical maneuvers that can be performed so as to help diagnose the symptoms as hysterical. The physician should be aware that individuals with genuine deafness have certain characteristics: 1. They speak in a monotonous voice with loud accentuations. 2. They usually watch the lips of the speakers. 3. They move their good ears towards the speaker. 4. Generally, vowels are heard better than consonants. Before examining a patient for deafness, the external ear must be cleared of wax and the tympanic membrane viewed. *All hearing tests should be performed with the patient blindfolded.* The Weber test should first be performed by having a vibrating tuning fork placed on the top of the head or on the glabella. Normally, the patient will perceive the vibration and sound in the midline or equally in both ears. If the patient has organic deafness due to obstruction of the conducting apparatus, i.e., middle ear disease, then the sound is heard louder and longer in the affected ear. However, when the deafness is due to nerve damage (cochlea or inner ear disease), the sound is heard stronger in the normal non-affected ear. The other test to be performed is the Rinné test. In this procedure, a normally placed vibrating tuning fork is placed behind the mastoid process and then in front of the ear, and air and bone conduction are compared. If air conduction is greater than bone conduction (normal occurrence), the test is considered positive. If bone conduction is greater than air conduction, the test is considered negative. By having a knowledge of these two tests, the clinician can now look for inconsistent patterns of "alleged deafness." With the patient blindfolded, several maneuvers can be performed:

1. By plugging the good ear with the finger, the examiner can ask the patient if he can still hear and if he answers, this indicates that hearing is present in the allegedly deaf ear.

2. One can place a tube into the "deaf ear" with an open lumen and then occlude the good ear with the finger and ask if he can hear. Again, if the patient answers affirmatively, then this indicates hysterical auditory loss.

3. The patient can be distracted by the physician with other events and then given a command; if he follows this request, hearing is present.

The *Lombard test* is a simple technique to detect unilateral deafness. The patient is asked to read aloud a specific paragraph and as long as he hears his own voice, there is no change in pitch. A specific Barany noise apparatus is inserted into the normal ear while the patient continues reading. If deafness is present, he will raise his voice. If he does not raise his voice, he probably hears with the allegedly deaf ear.

Another test for unilateral deafness is the *Bloch-Stenger test*, which is based on the physiological principle that, normally, when two vibrating tuning forks of different pitch are held simultaneously and equidistantly in front of both ears, only the one of higher pitch is audible. The examiner can test the allegedly deaf ear with a higher pitched fork to determine the responses.

Another test for unilateral deafness uses a stethoscope, the earplugs of which can be closed and adjusted to each ear. When the patient has the earplugs adjusted, one in each ear, the physician can speak into the bell of the stethoscope and ask the patient to repeat what he hears. Since the patient will be blindfolded, he will not know which side has been occluded and will respond erroneously.

When bilateral deafness occurs and hysteria is suspect, the demonstration of K-complexes in a sleep EEG confirm intact pathways (Fig. 19). Hysterical deafness also disappears during sleep. Consequently, an *unexpected* loud noise while the patient is asleep, may clarify the situation. In a well-documented case of hysterical deafness, Ventry describes audiological techniques that can successfully confirm the diagnosis.

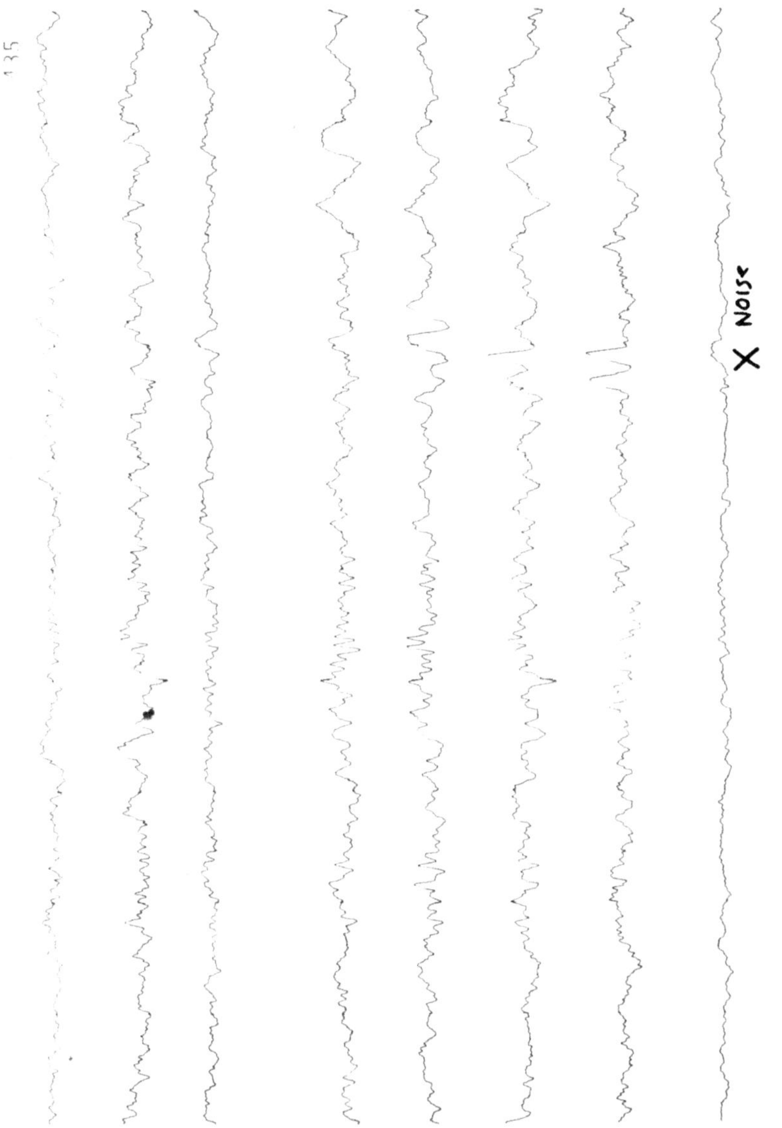

19 Demonstrates a cortical response (K-complex) to environmental noise.

Review of the literature indicates that hysterical deafness is usually a transitory symptom appearing suddenly in relation to a stressful event. It is usually associated with other focal hysterical symptoms such as blindness or loss of smell. Unusual dichotomy of symptoms may also be present such as deafness but intact musical perception, etc.

Head trauma is a common cause of concussion of the cochlea apparatus with resulting tinnitus and diminished hearing. Also, hysterical deafness can be seen under these identical circumstances making it quite difficult for the physician at times to determine the validity of symptoms.

Dizziness

Dizziness is a frequent complaint but true vertigo is only rarely hysterical in origin. Usually this is iatrogenically induced by the physician in his questioning of the patient. The symptom becomes refined into a true vertigo. The most common etiology for dizziness in the practice of medicine is the hyperventilation syndrome. The symptoms can be easily reproduced by asking the patient to voluntarily overventilate. There are many organic conditions that also have dizziness as a major symptom, including temporal lobe epilepsy, multiple sclerosis, labyrinthitis, brain tumor, cerebral concussion and cerebral ischemia. Consequently, this symptom requires careful evaluation and attention by the clinician.

Case: A thirty-six year old female had dizziness and syncope on three occasions within a month. Examination revealed a tense female with hyperactive deep tendon reflexes and a positive hyperventilation test. After the patient was reassured that no obvious organic lesion was lurking and that an emotional causation for her symptoms was most probable, she started to cry and said, "I have to tell somebody my problems." She had been having an affair with her friend's husband for several months. Now his job required his transfer to another part of the country. Her response to the anxiety of separation converted into hyperventilation, dizziness, and syncope as a means of avoiding making a decision on the matter.

True vertigo is often accompanied by nystagmus and autonomic symptoms of nausea, vomiting, sweating and pallor. The absence of these symptoms, however, is not inconsistent with the diagnosis of true vertigo. Since many organic conditions can produce vertigo, the clinician may require various specific tests including electronystagmography, Dix-Hallpike caloric testing, as well as CAT scan, spinal fluid analysis and possible angiography.

SPEECH DISORDERS

Speech disturbances are rarely hysterical in origin, but when they do occur, they can take the form of mutism and whispering speech (aphonia). The complaint occurs more frequently in children than in adults. The diagnosis can be more clearly defined by asking the patient to cough. If the cough is loud, it indicates that the vocal cords can be approximated and vagal nerve functions are normal. This can also be corroborated by direct visualization of the vocal cords (Fig. 20). If the patient has a true vocal cord paralysis and is requested to cough, a loud, booming bovine sound is heard. In addition, his voice is also affected. Thus, the simple cough test will clearly distinguish between hysteria and organic symptoms. Observation of palatal movements is also helpful. Hysterical aphonia occurs less frequently than mutism and indicates less negative and oppositional aspects in the patient's personality. It usually arises suddenly after an emotional crisis. An interesting example occurred in 1933 when a famous actress was grazed negligently by a collapsing stage curtain. There was no evidence of bodily injury but she developed a hysterical aphonia. The actress received a jury verdict of $50,000. Within two years of the settlement, the actress had fully recovered her voice and was giving concerts.

Hysterical mutism indicates a more serious personality problem with extreme negativism. These patients usually do not make any effort to move the lips or tongue or raise the soft palate. They act as if they do not hear or understand, yet they can read and write. These patients must be differentiated from those with expressive aphasia of Broca (Broddman's area 44), which usually accompanies a stroke. These organic patients are visibly upset in their inability to speak and become quite emotional. Other organic conditions producing mutism include akinetic mutism and tumors. Abnormal examination findings are usually present in underlying organic etiology.

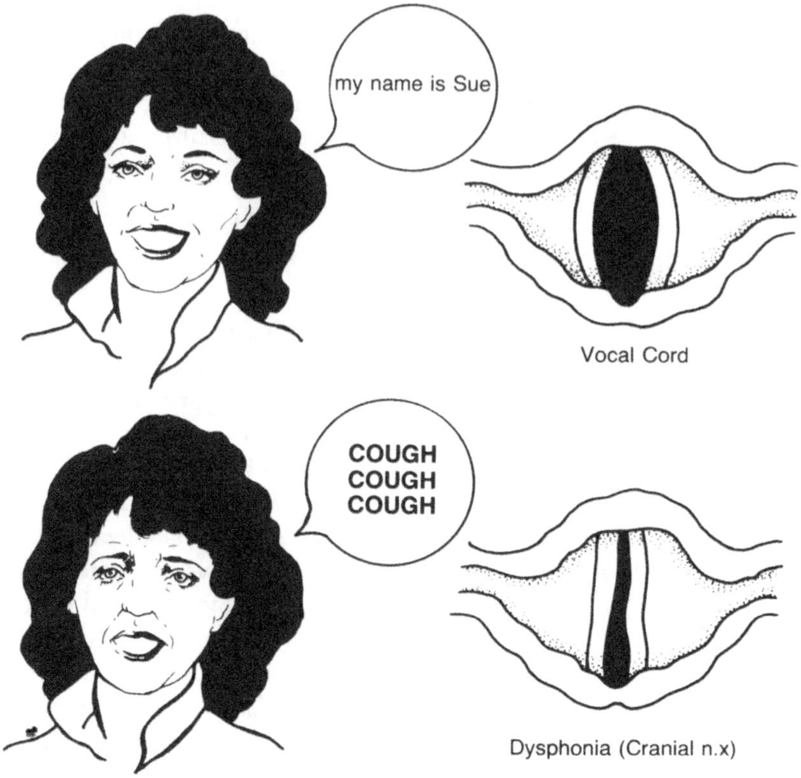

20 Cough test and vagal nerve function.

A recent article by Kalman and Graven demonstrates the usefulness of the written interview in hysterical mutism. Review of the literature reveals that hysterical mutism usually disappears as quickly as it arises. Consequently, numerous therapies have been employed. These include hypnosis, suggestion, amytal interview, faradic stimulation of the vocal cords, voice exercises, speech therapy and psychotherapy-psychoanalysis.

Case: A 15 year old problem student was caught stealing. He could not speak but could write answers to questions. After a period of time and with supportive environment, he was able to handle his situation emotionally and began to speak.

SWALLOWING DISTURBANCES

The syndrome of *globus hystericus* refers to the common swallowing difficulties that produce a "lump" in the throat and choking sensation (Fig. 21). It is often an intermittent, painful syndrome that does not permit easy swallowing of liquids or solid foods. The patients tend to have these as chronic symptoms and a barium swallow esophagram and upper GI series are invariably performed. Palatal and swallowing disturbances caused by glossopharyngeal and vagal nerve dysfunction (organic etiologies) rarely produce "lump in throat feeling" and are rarely accompanied by pain. This fact helps to distinguish it from the globus reaction.

One of my ENT colleagues, Dr. Gerald Rosmarin, has achieved almost 100% successful results in treating these patients with Hurst dilatation. When he is convinced that no other possible organic pathology exists and reassurance and/or tranquilizer are ineffective, he usually advises dilatation. The patient is met in the morning N.P.O. and usually started with swallowing a #28 dilator. Depending on the ease of the maneuver, he may progress at either two or four size increments to a #40 dilator. He does not pass the dilator beyond the mid-esophagus, and on followup examination, the tightness and/or lump sensation is completely reversed.

Glossopharyngeal neuralgia has a characteristic focality and localization with a triggering influence. The use of topical anesthetics or Tegretol are quite useful in this rare neuralgia.

Case: I recently examined a young woman with a three month history of dysphagia. This was intermittent and unrelated to the type (solid or liquid) or amount of food ingested. There was no nausea or emesis and a screening neurological examination and upper GI series were normal. Inquiry into her social background revealed that prior to the onset of symptoms, she was having an affair and practiced fellatio which, in retrospect, she felt to be disgusting. When she realized this association, her symptoms promptly disappeared.

Other hysterical gastrointestinal symptoms can be seen in people of all ages. Characteristically, children develop aerophagia with abdominal distention.

Hysterical women who have an intense desire to be pregnant develop the condition of pseudocyesis. The abdominal protuberance is brought about by simultaneously relaxing the abdominal

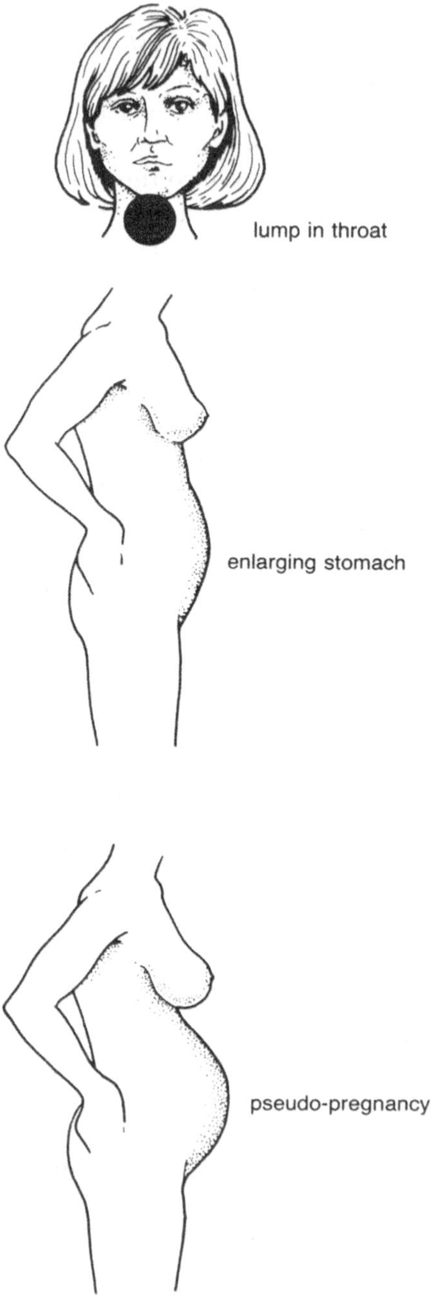

21 Hysterical syndromes: globus hystericus, aerophagia, pseudocyeisis.

muscles and thrusting the lumbar spine (Fig. 21). Cultural influences were recently discussed by Lapido in the infertile Nigerian female. It appears there is a high premium on childbearing as well as the cultural belief that children are "security" for old age. These cultural influences thereby expose these infertile females to constant stress. Thus, social, economic and psychological influences beset this specific culture in which there is a high incidence of pseudocyesis.

Psychogenic vomiting is a frequent syndrome presenting to the primary care physician, internist and gastroenterologist. Typically, these patients link their symptoms closely with environmental stress. They are usually not incapacitated or seriously impaired. In a review of twenty-four such patients, Rosenthal and co-workers found that most of their patients disliked confrontation and disagreement, and vomiting seemed to resolve their conflict by symbolically purging their anger. Some patients were depressed but the majority did not have serious psychiatric disturbances and were not incapacitated by their illness. The vomiting tended to be chronic.

A more dramatic syndrome, anorexia nervosa, often classified as a hysterical conversion reaction, results as a consequence of complex interaction of psychologic abnormalities, endocrine disturbances, and malnutrition. Although a spectrum of psychological disorders have been observed, distortion of body image, weight phobia from a disordered perception of hunger and satiety, the illness is considered a bio-psychological disorder. It is felt that multiple factors interact in a vulnerable person producing marked self-induced weight loss, psychological changes and secondary physiological abnormalities. There is controversy as to whether anorexia nervosa is a disease entity or a symptom complex occurring in persons with diverse psychopathology. Sir William Gull in an address at Oxford in 1868, discussed this condition as "hysteric apepsia" and later coined the term, "anorexia hysterica" and ultimately, "anorexia nervosa." Freud considered this a neurosis in pubescent girls who symbolically were expressing aversion to sexuality by means of anorexia and fear of all impregnation or attempts at seduction. Many other explanations have been offered by patients as well as physicians but in a significant majority of these individuals, body image distortion is found. Lucas recently reviewed this controversial topic.

Other hysterical abdominal complaints include appendicitis, hiccupping and sneezing.

ALTERATIONS OF CONSCIOUSNESS—PSYCHOGENIC SEIZURES

One of the most perplexing and difficult diagnoses confronting the physician is the hysterical seizure or pseudoseizure. This event is usually not witnessed by a physician and, therefore, the patient is usually asymptomatic. Nonetheless, an aggressive organic workup must be vigorously pursued. It is often argued that hysterical fits are uncommon (Laidlaw and Richens) despite the classical description of hystero-epilepsy made by Charcot. Other authors find hysterical fits to be common (Riley and Massey). Ljungberg found hysterical convulsions to be the second most common conversion syndrome, accounting for 20% of his cases. Grand mal movements are more often simulated than focal Jacksonian motor contractions, petit mal or psychomotor disturbances. At the onset, hysterical convulsions are defined as a subjective loss of consciousness without ictal discharges in response to psychological stimuli. Usually these are daytime occurrences without any evidence of external injury arising. There is no tongue biting, urinary incontinence or tonic clonic movements of cerebral origin. Usually these attacks occur in front of a large audience. The duration of these attacks is usually from fifteen to thirty minutes. The deep tendon reflexes are present without Babinski response. In order for the clinician to confirm the diagnosis, he must be able to distinguish hysterical convulsions from true epilepsy. This may be somewhat difficult. The major practical aspect of this problem encountered in practice is that pseudoseizures usually occur in patients manifesting a true epileptic disorder. Secondary gains may be obvious. Those patients who are quite experienced or knowledgeable about epilepsy can enhance their presentation accordingly. An occurrence of 10–20% in out-patient Epileptic populations has been recognized. In addition, since epilepsy is a common disorder and is frequently seen on television, most individuals have achieved a degree of familiarity with this sympton.

The relationship between epilepsy and hysteria often poses a diagnostic challenge to the physician. The recognition of a specific pseudoseizure is not easy due to a lack of absolute criteria. It has been suggested that blood prolactin levels, under these circumstances, may be informative and diagnostic since they tend to rise after a "true" epileptic seizure but not after a psychogenic seizure. I do not believe this to be a valid observation and the assay

TABLE 6.
Organic vs. Hysterical Signs

Loss of consciousness
Babinski response
Post-ictal stupor

is often fraught with error. One must recognize that the issue is quite complex. It has been suggested that ten percent of intractable convulsions have a psychogenic origin and are often mistakenly treated with anti-epileptic drugs. The experienced physician may be able to clarify the confusion by observing the bizarre sequences of movements and contortions that bear little resemblance to the true tonic-clonic movements of grand mal epilepsy. Many of the movements resemble the sex act. Clonic jerking of various extremities, without tonic movement or loss of consciousness are the rule. These "seizures" can last from minutes to hours and in many cases can be influenced by suggestion. As a generalization during these spells, hysterical patients do not lose consciousness and do not injure themselves. They do not manifest the epileptic shrill or cry, tongue biting or urinary incontinence, nor do they have post-ictal stupor. However on rare occasions they may be present. Characteristically, these episodes are spectacular performances in front of a large audience, and on some occasions observers are bitten by the patient. Examination of the patient during this spell, if possible (Table 6), would reveal no loss of consciousness, intact corneal reflex, and no Babinski. On occasion, the motor activity is aggravated with attempts at restraint. An EEG, if performed, would not demonstrate epileptiform activity producing the above attack (Fig. 26). Table 6 helps to clarify the distinction between these two conditions. To compound the

TABLE 7.
Parietal Lobe Dysfunction

1. Tactile inattention
2. Visual inattention
3. Cortical sensory loss
4. Hemianesthesia
5. Pseudothalamic syndrome
6. Pseudoathetosis
7. Hemiatrophy
8. Constructional apraxia

problem for the physician who is witnessing such an attack, these symptoms often occur in patients with a true convulsive disorder and, thus, the aspects of primary and secondary gains become important and relevant in this situation. I find sternal massage during the actual spell to be a valuable test in determining organicity. Deep, sustained pressure will not alter a true grand mal seizure but the unpleasant sensation will disturb hysterics and they will attempt to push the hand away or grab it to make it stop. One's experience in observing verified epileptic seizures proves an invaluable guide in deciding whether such spells are organic or hysterical and deserving of therapy. This point is extremely important. Once a flurry of "convulsions" is considered organic, patients are given large amounts of parenteral medications, i.e., phenobarbital, Valium, Dilantin and subcutaneous paraldehyde. The patient will, of course, become sedated and may have respiratory embarrassment. In addition, primary and secondary gains are reinforced with this augmented attention.

Case: A 46 year old male schizophrenic with a true seizure disorder was hospitalized on the psychiatric floor with three roommates in a buddy system where all members tried to help each other. The patient went into a "spell" one evening and thrashed about. Two roommates went for the hospital staff and one remained with the patient. After a few minutes, I arrived and observed the writhing movements. There was no Babinski and corneal reflexes were present. Firm sternal massage brought a major response with the patient grabbing my hand and stating, "That hurts."

Case: A thirty-five year old male with true and hysterical convulsions was hospitalized for observation as he was under a moderate emotional strain. Several hysterical convulsions were observed and, consequently, the staff was alerted. On one occasion, his roommate ran for the nurse because the patient had been shaking unresponsively for five minutes. The nurse looked in, saw the patient "jerking" and walked away. The patient, seeing this, stopped his movements and yelled to the nurse that she was not interested in caring for him.

A word of caution is required at this point especially for those treating patients with temporal lobe (limbic) epilepsy. Bizarre behavioral alterations including automatisms, subjective experiences and fugue may be seen frequently and these are usually due to the disease process with elements of interictal psychosis. Figs. 22, 23, 24, 25 demonstrate various EEG patterns of epilepsy. Many of these patients find themselves in trouble with the law and it is difficult for the physician to state emphatically that their "misbehavior" was due to the seizure rather than premeditated. During the majority of episodes, the patient is not completely aware of the events. Telemetric electroencephalography and video monitoring have helped differentiate epileptic from non-epileptic attacks, whereas an inter-seizure EEG is unreliable. In an excellent study by Binnie and co-workers, it was demonstrated that experienced neurologists who diagnosed certain convulsions as psychogenic turned out to be wrong, as these represented true epileptic events. They described a specific case of a young woman with many psychosocial problems who would, from time to time, lower her head and wrap her hands about her body and shake her head from side to side. An attack occurred during monitoring and proved to be a seizure of temporal lobe origin. Other investigators have found as many as 36% recorded pseudoseizures and these had a greater tendency to occur during the first recording session. Diagnosis was determined by assessment of four major criteria: 1. deviation of seizures from characteristics of known seizure types, 2. absence of epileptiform activity in the ictal EEG, 3. absence of slowing in the post-ictal EEG, and 4. relation of seizure frequency to decreasing plasma concentration of anti-epileptic drugs.

The diagnosis of hysterical attacks may be difficult even with prolonged monitoring and it has been suggested that a standardized "provocative" saline infusion be used, associated with the suggestion that an attack will occur and then will stop. Cohen and Suter demonstrated this method in 41 patients and found it to be reproducible and accurate. However it must be recognized that patients with a chronic illness such as epilepsy are often dependent and suggestible, and wish to please their physicians. Complicating the issue further is the fact that a high percentage of patients with pseudoseizures have abnormal electroencephalograms; this suggests some central nervous system abnormality. Standage, in a major review, found this to be present in forty percent of cases. His experience indicates that epileptic seizures and pseudo-seizures are in no way incompatible and most neurologists believe that these patients should be treated by both anticonvulsants and

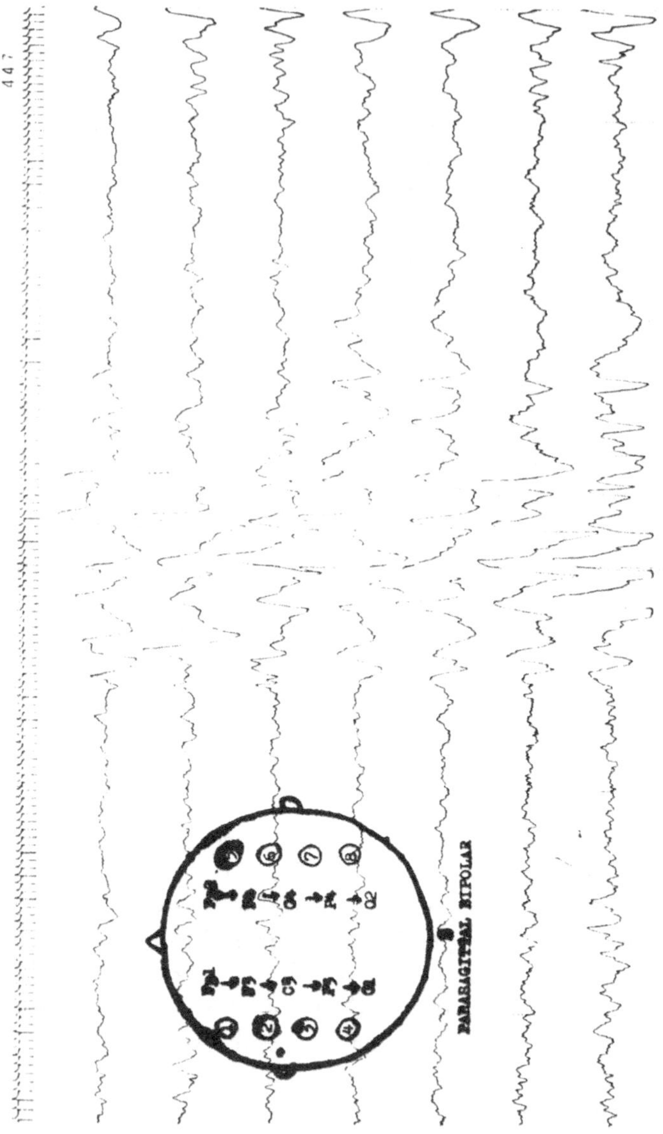

22 Demonstrates paroxysomal epileptic burst in response to photic stimulation. The patient manifested grand mal epilepsy.

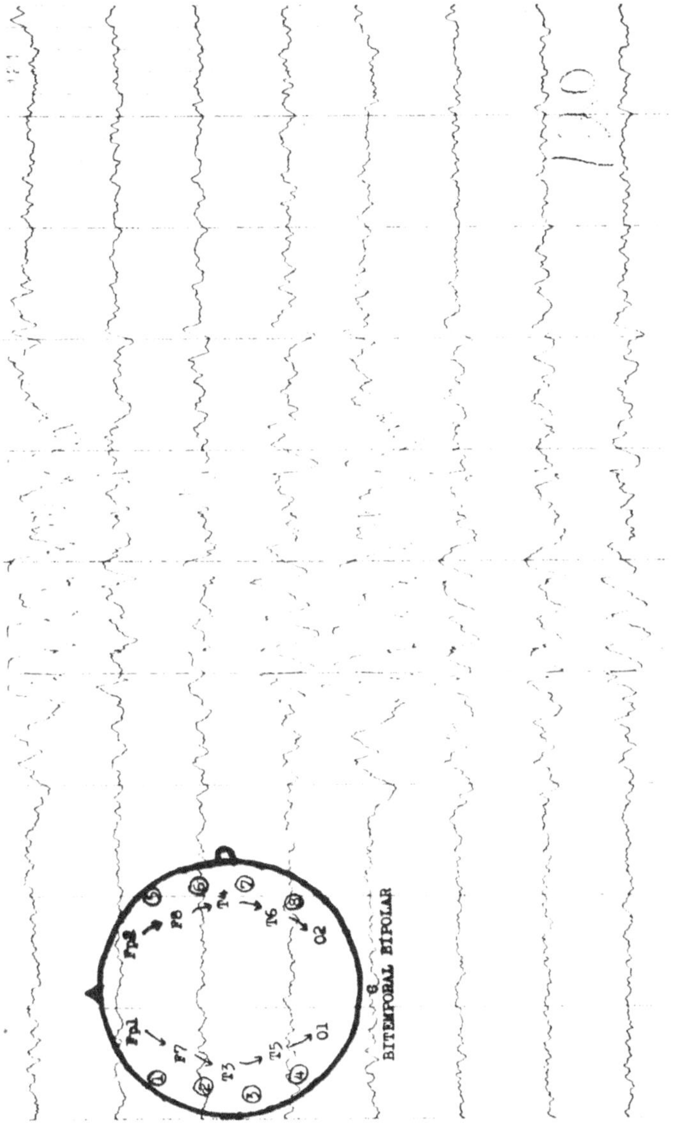

23 Epileptic response (spike and wave) to hyperventilation maneuver. Unusual staring and isolated jerks were seen in association with these discharges.

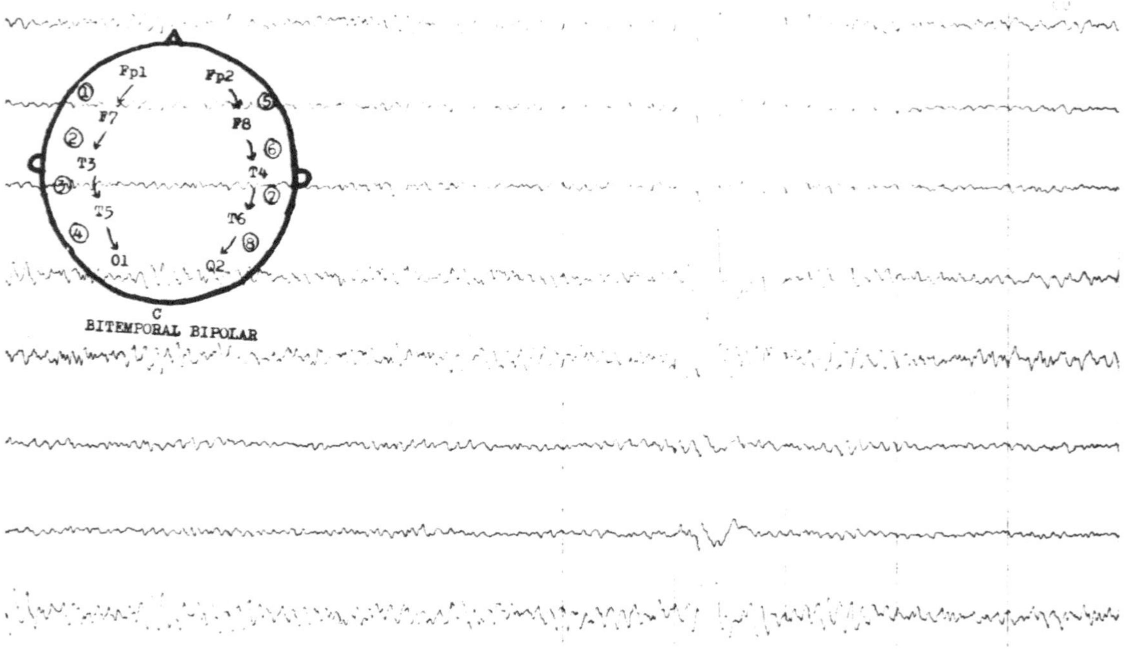

24 Isolated epileptiform burst in patient manifesting functional sensory changes on examination but complaining of headache relating to another accident.

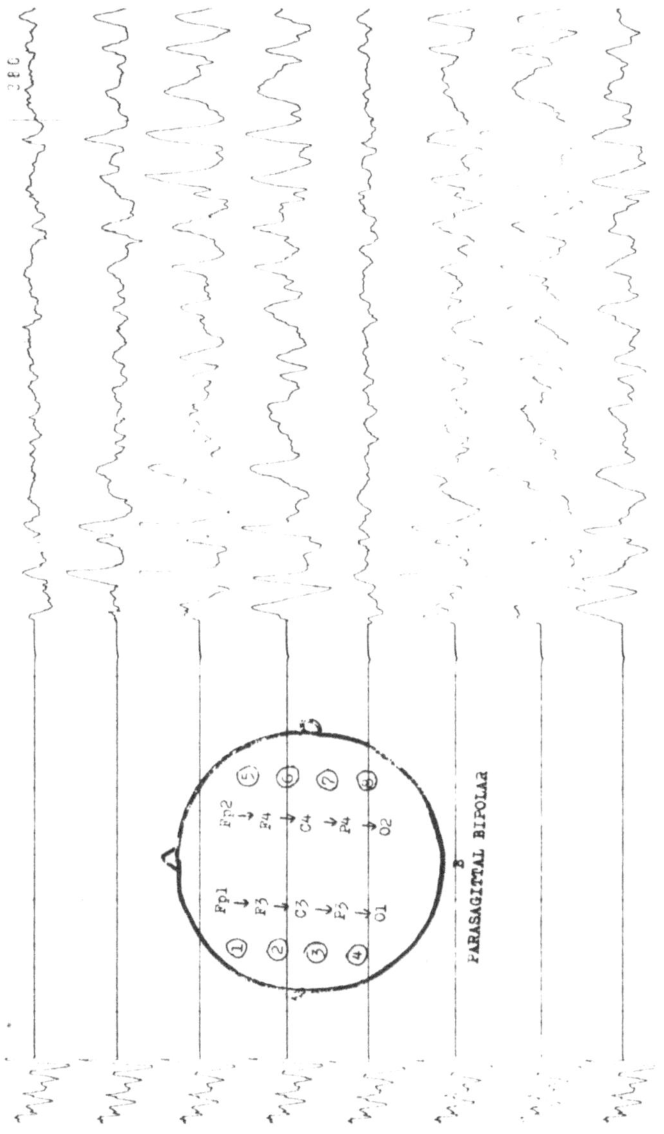

25 Patient always appears "dazed" with suggestion of underlying psychiatric illness. Note excessive spike-wave discharges (temporal lobe epilepsy).

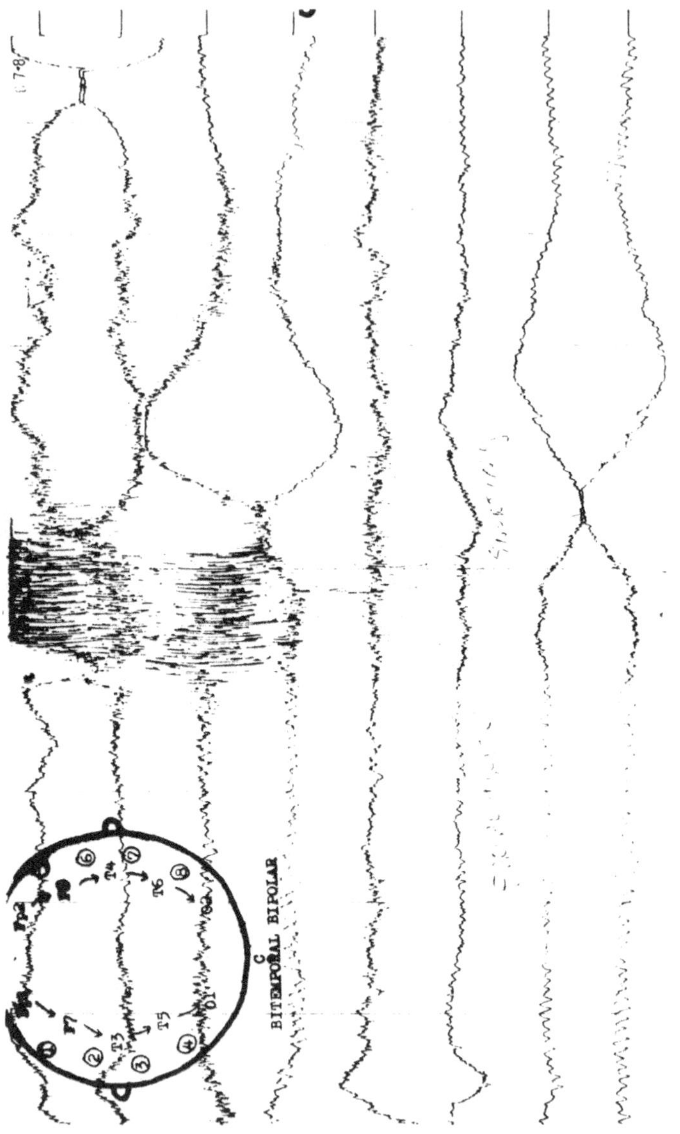

26 Psychogenic seizure with bizarre facial contortions and snorting. No cortical epileptiform discharges developed. Note excess muscle movement artifact during this activity.

psychiatric treatment. EEG telemetry appears to be the best test. Neuropsychological performance tests have not clarified the problem although it has been suggested by Sackellares, et al., that performance tests are better predictors of organicity.

It should be noted that many epileptic phenomena have been confused with psychiatric disease, particularly schizophrenia. Temporal lobe automatisms with interictal psychosis and petit mal status, which can last for several days, may also complicate the diagnosis. Anticonvulsants can play some role, in that they modify the epileptic activity so that bizarre equivalents may be present. In a series of 666 patients with temporal lobe epilepsy and on drugs, 17 patients had gross hysterical disorders such as ataxia and paralysis (Currie et al.).

Clinical evidence suggests that acute emotional stress is an important factor in precipitating epileptic convulsions and hysterical seizures. It is clear that in many of these patients, sexual traumata are a factor. Historically, Galen believed that the hysterical seizures were the result of premature intercourse in childhood and Freud believed that hysterical convulsions represented a traumatic event. A growing list of studies demonstrates hysterical convulsions to be a sequel to incest. Goodwin described six cases of Navajo folklore connecting epilepsy with incest and bewitchment. All six patients experienced relief from the hysterical symptoms when psychotherapy discovered the hidden incestuous relationship. In this review, he found a ten percent incidence of hysterical conversion convulsions associated with prior incest. LaBarbera and Dozier described four adolescent cases of hysterical seizures immediately preceded by some event that was overtly sexual or that was construed as having sexual meaning.

Dissociative experiences such as fugue with or without amnesia, multiple personalities, hallucinations, demoniacal possession are often attributed to psychiatric disease, yet these symptoms often fall into the borderlands of neurology and psychiatry. Although the etiological mechanisms remain controversial, a significant number of cases have abnormal temporal lobe discharges on electroencephalograms as illustrated in the twelve cases of Mesulan. Each of the patients was initially seen by psychiatrists and a diagnosis of hysteria was made in three. Two cases had a diagnosis of schizophrenia. He demonstrated that dissociative phenomena were more common from the non-dominant hemisphere.

FUGUE STATES AND AMNESIA

Fugue states are altered states of consciousness with varying degrees of motor activity and amnesia. They present a perplexing diagnostic challenge because of the vagueness of the terminology. Two clinical entities that must be considered from the organic standpoint are transient global amnesia and migraine. An excellent review by Akhtar and Brenner helped to clarify the differential diagnosis of these states. Their main conclusions are that a complete history, physical exam and neurological workup, including a lumbar puncture, CAT scan, EEG with nasopharyngeal leads and even an amytal interview may be necessary to clarify the issue. It is commonly believed that these alterations are temporally related to psychological stress. These diagnostic divisions are clearly fraught with error, even in experienced hands. Recently, Gross demonstrated an incorrect diagnosis of epilepsy in thirteen adolescent patients with hysterical seizures and amnesic fugues, who were treated with anticonvulsants an average of 15.5 months before the correct diagnosis was made.

Another common hysterical alteration of consciousness is conversion syncope seen in young girls and women. Typically, the faint occurs in the presence of others and lasts only seconds to minutes. During the actual faint, there are no changes in the vital signs, color and sweating, and the patient can be observed to be hyperventilating. Thus, for the physician evaluating cases of syncope or dizziness, the hyperventilation test is quite a useful tool in duplicating the symptoms (Fig. 27). The precipitating influence may be suddenly identified or else the patient may suffer from periodic panic or anxiety attacks. Typically, the patient feels a surging build-up of tension and anxiety followed by overbreathing. The patient is usually unaware of this hyperventilation. This maneuver quickly changes the oxygen/carbon dioxide ratio producing elements of cerebral ischemia and hypoxia leading to lightheadedness, paresthesiae of lips and digits and, ultimately, tetany. If the overbreathing continues, syncope may occur. The distinction from epilepsy must be made carefully since epileptic attacks may be produced by anxiety and/or over-ventilation and

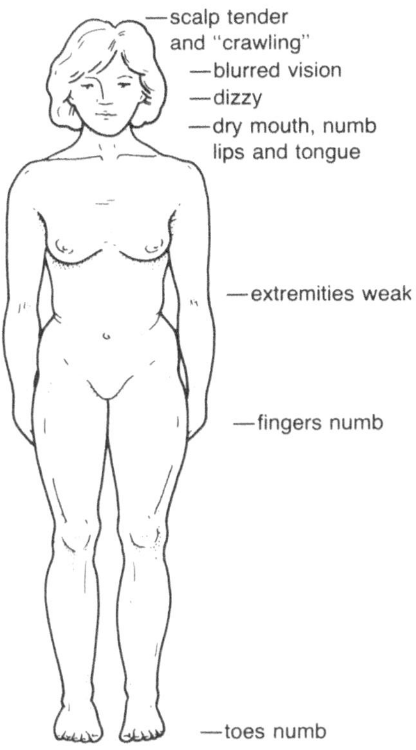

27 Hyperventilation syndrome.

this is the basis for the provocative hyperventilation test during the performance of the standard electroencephalogram. Observation of the patient during the episode will usually clarify the diagnosis because true epileptic seizures are not present.

Hysterical coma is an extension of syncope and often resembles the organic condition of akinetic mutism. However, upon closer examination, the pupils and corneal reflexes are active and the plantar reflexes are flexor. Active resistance by the patient often occurs when the physician attempts to examine. Psychogenic coma may be differentiated from organic coma by the use of cold caloric stimulation. Irrigation of the ear with ten milliliters of ice water induces a normal, rapid phase of nystagmus to the *opposite* side in HCR whereas there is an *ipsilateral nystagmus* in true coma (with intact brainstem).

Hysterical amnesia appears in a variety of guises and is a frequent clinical disturbance. The diagnosis can be made easily if the patient retains the ability to eat, dress, speak and read, yet denies his personal identity. Since acquired learned behavior is lost early in organic dysfunction, the opposite should prevail.

Hysterical dementia was first described by Ganser in 1898 and consists of the syndrome of approximate answers. This is almost always seen in incarcerated males. Parietal lobe disorders may be confused with hysterical conversion reactions because they are so bizarre. Common clinical presentations include the following (Table 7): 1. tactile inattention (extinction, 2. visual inattention (extinction), 3. cortical sensory loss, 4. hemianesthesia, 5. pseudothalamic syndrome, 6. pseudoathetosis, 7. hemiatrophy, and 8. construction apraxia. It is only by awareness of the above presentations that the clinician will avoid an error in diagnosis.

There has been a mistaken notion that patients diagnosed as suffering from hysteria are less likely to commit suicide than patients with affective disorders. In recent longterm studies, both Lester and Guze have demonstrated an equally great risk (15%) in both groups. Therefore, the physician must be vigilant when patients express suicidal ideation.

7

CHILDHOOD CONVERSION REACTIONS

Hysteria in childhood requires a separate section due to the different manifestations and psychodynamic mechanisms involved. More importantly, its frequent occurrence has escaped significant appreciation by physicians. For those clinicians caring for young children, the importance of oral mechanisms tends to be more obvious than genital fixations. However, as children get older and more mature the latter assumes greater importance.

Several standard pediatric textbooks and older examples of the literature indicate that the onset of hysterical conversion reactions before the age of ten is rare. I feel that this statement is erroneous and requires modification since:

1. There is semantic confusion about the term hysteria.
2. Previous studies were only on hospitalized patients and the results are open to various interpretations.
3. Reports are almost exclusively from psychiatrists rather than other physicians who see a wider spectrum of pediatric and adolescent illness.
4. Clinical observations suggest a higher incidence.

A recent report by Schneider and Rice of a pediatric neurology in-patient population, found a 2% incidence over a 4½ year time period and these authors concluded that hysteria is far more common than generally appreciated. This study is also significant in demonstrating that no referring physician ever suggested the diagnosis of hysterical conversion reaction as possibly causing the neurological symptoms. Thus, neurological symptoms of hysterical conversion reaction are infrequently recognized by pediatricians and family physicians. These authors speculated that many children with suspected chronic neurological disease, especially epilepsy, may in reality have a chronic hysterical conversion reaction.

The criteria for the diagnosis of hysterical conversion reaction in children should be the same as that for adults — namely, positive evidence from the clinical examination. The symptoms must not conform to known neuroanatomy or physiology. In addition, a significant relationship of the symptoms to a recent emotional crisis can usually be demonstrated. The type of symptoms manifested depend on maturity, intelligence, experience and cultural influence. Consequently, one observes simple and primitive conversion reactions in a young child and complex conversion reactions in an adolescent. An additional part of the examination that may be useful in children is the use of drawings. Chenven recently reported that children with HCR may draw pictures of themselves with distortions in the "afflicted" body part. He described some children with hysterical paraplegia drawing patients with absent or distorted legs. Similarly, alterations in head anatomy were noted in some children with conversion headaches.

INCIDENCE OF HYSTERIA IN CHILDREN

It is difficult to arrive at a fixed percentage but I suspect that at least 5% of the pediatric population may have hysterical conversion reactions before they reach adulthood. Personal experience convinces me that these conversions are often overlooked in the differential diagnosis of neurological symptoms in children, and the reports of Schneider and Rice confirm my observation. The onset of symptoms may be abrupt or gradual. Typically, the symptoms are precipitated by a unique emotional experience, such as divorce of parents, death in the family, or injury. Hospitalization often will occur during the acute phase of illness. In children below age ten, the ratio of females and males is approximately equal, but by the adolescent years, females constitute the bulk of patients.

The symptoms seen are usually multiple and roughly parallel those occurring in adults. Specific aspects of these presentations will be discussed.

SENSORY DISTURBANCES

The wide variety of sensory disturbances in adults described above also apply to children. Sensory mapping, which demonstrates sharply demarcated borders that do not follow dermatomal patterns or fail to cross the midline, are good clues and indicate the patient's own naive concept of body anatomy. Patients also complain of isolated concentric areas of sensory loss. The abdomen and joints seem to be the areas of predisposition and pain is more frequent than anesthesia. At times, suggestion can alter the intensity and distribution of these symptoms quite dramatically. The common belly pain in the young and school-aged individual raises questions of appendicitis, intestinal obstruction or even malignancy, especially when the symptoms become chronic or intense. Many of these children show immaturity and marked dependency needs. Some, coming from achievement-oriented homes, are fearful of failure.

MOTOR DISTURBANCES

Motor manifestations in children are equally variable but less dramatic than in adults. They include grimacing, head shaking, head banging, throat clearing, sniffing, shrugging of the shoulders, wrinkling of the forehead, gaping, and eye blinking. All of these movements can be considered under the term "tics." These are extremely common occurrences in young children. They often tend to be ignored until they interfere with social or learning processes. These movements are performed suddenly, quickly and repetitively, and usually last for a few months. Most tics in children appear between the ages of seven and ten, last a few months, and then disappear. A small minority of tics persist into adolescence and adulthood. The physician must consider several organic diseases in children with such tics, including Wilson's disease, Sydenham's chorea, Gilles de la Tourette's syndrome, and degenerative basal ganglionic disease of childhood, before determining these to be purely psychological symptoms. It is believed that the individuals are under extreme emotional tension and are attempting to free themselves of their dependent needs within the family situation. Tics are rarely observed in relaxed and non-pressured family situations.

Another common presentation is motor weakness in an extremity with the development of a limp, a spastic contracture (Gold; Ehrlich and Fisher) or gait disturbance. Usually, these children have previously observed a person with such a disability. Part of the psychological background of some children involves fear of failing at a specific motor task.

Tremor of the extremities is common, and varies in duration and extent. Observations during play or eating help in diagnosis. Scoliosis and torticollis are other motor alterations. The clinician must remain alert to the possibility of a congenital diaphragmatic defect with hiatus hernia as an etiology for torticollis and body posturing. This is called Sandifer's syndrome and is a well-defined clinical entity in young children due to hiatus hernia with gastroesophageal reflux. These children, in attempting to prevent aspiration, assume bizarre body postures. It is felt that these children are manifesting a primary neurological disease of brainstem or cerebellar pathways. This unappreciated entity has been discussed recently by Werlin.

A significant number of children come to the pediatrician or family practitioner with "unexplained" vomiting, diarrhea, constipation, hiccups, difficulty opening the mouth, *globus hystericus* and aerophagia. If the symptoms become protracted, the physician is ultimately forced to perform several radiological procedures such as a gastrointestinal series or esophagogram. Questions asked of family members usually shed light on a recent "crisis" in the family such as the birth of another child, death of a family member or arguments. Maloney recently reported a higher frequency of recent family stress (97%), unresolved grief reactions (58%), and family communication problems (77%) in children with HCR compared to controls. These children tend to have multiple visceral complaints in response to stress. It is imperative for the family practitioner and pediatrician to develop techniques for questioning for psychological stress and adaptive responses, as they may be able to unravel those unconscious feelings of the patient and thereby aid in certain personality readjustments. Only by this active intervention can one hope to reduce the chronicity of visceral complaints. It is of interest to note that children of physicians tend to be more "bodily oriented" than other children and visceral symptoms tend to be a major complaint.

CRANIAL NERVE DISTURBANCES

Visual alterations are frequent complaints and take many forms. Blurring and image distortion are perhaps the most frequent complaints. While migraine is the most frequent disease producing this symptom, it is singularly unusual without other concomitant features. A positive family history, as well as headache and autonomic changes, should be looked for. Intrinsic ocular disease must also be ruled out. The pupillary response is, indeed, important in this determination. *Blindness* is an extension of the above visual symptoms and again, the principles discussed in the adult section apply. Yasuna reported twenty-six cases of hysterical amblyopia in children nine to fourteen years of age. Seventy-five percent were in girls and the condition was principally bilateral. These patients demonstrated no difficulty in moving about a room and the individuals did not bump into objects or handle objects like an organically blind person.

In general, most children complaining of hysterical visual alterations have diverse psychiatric problems; these symptoms tend to prevent them from performing a task at which they subconsciously feel they will fail.

Monocular diplopia is not infrequently seen. The inexperienced pediatrician or family practitioner will naturally consider a posterior fossa neoplasm in any child with this complaint. The examination of the eye will quickly rule out a detached retina and dislocated lens which organically can produce this condition. The red lens cover test will help clarify the complaint and demonstrate the false image if organic. I have observed this complaint in a neurologist's daughter. It can also be argued that the symptoms of double vision may be induced by the physician's questions. The same applies for vertigo.

Blepharospasm may be seen by itself or in association with tics. *Convergence spasm* is also a frequent presentation mimicking a bilateral abducens nerve palsy. Again, observation of pupillary responses and optokinetic nystagmus will help to clarify the diagnosis.

Hysterical deafness is usually observed in people who are afraid of failing in a specific task and who come from achievement-oriented families. Several young aviators who were faced with the prospect of death reacted with hysterical deafness. This deafness is not complete and disappears during sleep.

K-complexes can be observed on sleep electroencephalograms in response to sound thereby indicating intact auditory pathways. The major organic illness that must be distinguished from the above is childhood autism. Autistic children manifest a constellation of symptoms with primary disregard of humans. There is no eye contact or socialization and they are unable to be disciplined. Rarely does a central nervous system lesion produce *bilateral* deafness due to the multiple crossings of the auditory fibers in the trapezoid body and from the cochlea nucleus.

Dizziness is a frequent childhood symptom that may reflect hyperventilation, otitis media, otitis interna, migraine, temporal lobe epilepsy, benign paroxysmal vertigo of Barany, or, rarely, posterior fossa neoplasm. Only by a thorough examination with appropriate laboratory tests including the EEG and CAT scan, will the physician accurately arrive at the correct diagnosis. Hyperventilation is perhaps the most common syndrome producing this symptom and if it becomes extreme, syncope and tetany may develop. An interesting epidemic of hysterical conversion reactions was reported by Knight *et al.* in a group of adolescent Louisiana school children. This outbreak began when a rumor spread through the school that all the girls were to be tested for pregnancy and those with positive tests would be sent to a correctional school. Most of the students displayed the entire spectrum of hyperventilation with rapid breathing, dizziness, paresthesia, tremor and syncope. Twenty-one girls and one boy were affected.

HYSTERICAL COMA

Hysterical coma is rare but can be seen in extremely frightened children who have a rigid super-ego. From an organic standpoint, a drug overdose, convulsions, intracranial hemorrhage or infection are the major considerations to be ruled out. A careful neurological examination and several laboratory tests including an EEG, CAT scan, toxicology screen, lumbar puncture and glucose level, will quickly clarify the issue.

PSEUDOSEIZURES

Pseudoseizures constituted the largest number of patients

seen in the study by Schneider and Rice. Parents' descriptions of these spells differ from the careful observations of physicians. In most patients, the diagnosis was complicated and required serial evaluations over a few months before the actual definitive diagnosis could be established. As a rule, these children do not injure themselves nor do they demonstrate post-ictal confusion or EEG slowing. However, as previously mentioned in the adult section, recent data using telemetric monitoring has demonstrated bizarre temporal lobe discharges in otherwise "hysterical spells." Thus, many patients have a combination of true and hysterical seizures and thereby complicate the problem even further from a management standpoint.

DISSOCIATIVE/DEPERSONALIZATION REACTIONS

Sudden *amnesia* without head trauma or convulsions is not uncommon in children who are overwhelmed by anxiety. Again, their ability to eat, tie the shoes, and dress despite their selective loss of memory for name, address and telephone number clears up any question as to diagnosis. Likewise, the fugue-twilight state blends with the above to include a selective impairment. An EEG is useful in ruling out temporal lobe (limbic) epilepsy in over 90% of cases.

Nightmares and *sleepwalking* can be of epileptiform nature and most times, will leave the patient confused. They may have a vague dream-like remembrance of events or be totally amnestic of the event. However, in hysterical nightmares and sleepwalking, the patients "awaken" from the spell alert, passive and not frightened. Again, this is a generalization.

THERAPEUTIC COMMENTS

Hysterical conversion reaction in children, as in adults, reveals that a majority of these patients are immature and have extreme dependency needs. Other than this, no characteristic pattern emerges from an analysis of the literature or from personal experience. Psychologic and social maladjustments are not peculiar to the patient with hysterical conversion reaction. Thus, probing into personal problems is unreliable as an attempt to diagnose hysteria. The only criteria that is reproducible is the positive demonstration of findings that do not conform to anatomical and physiological principles. The standard methods of clinical medicine should prevail with accurate history of the presenting illness. Past and family history, educational background and schoolwork records are also reviewed, as well as the physical examination so that the clinician gets "the feel" of the case. If the patient is able to fully cooperate, this aspect may be a beneficial therapeutic experience. By following this therapeutic approach and demonstrating positive criteria from the examination, the physician should have a reasonably clear understanding of the basic problem and its psycho-dynamics. That these criteria and methods are not being carefully followed is surmised from the report of Forbis and James. These authors found a marked incidence of hysterical conversion reaction in children in Arkansas. To their surprise they found that many non-psychiatric physicians did not make the diagnosis. I suspect that their observations sixteen years ago are basically true today in many areas of the country. This point is also emphasized in the report by Schneider and Rice. On the other hand, clinicians must strongly suspect organic disease when "apparent" hysterical symptoms are found in an individual who is felt to have an intact personality structure.

Once the diagnosis of hysteria is established, treatment must be considered. Children differ from adults in that a total program is necessary. Parents must be handled in a positive manner that will help them accept the fact that the illness is emotional and not physical. Parents must be taught to assist their children by providing security and allowing emotional growth, thus improving the parent-child relationship. After this is accomplished, the children are relieved of their symptoms by any of several means (i.e., suggestion, hypnosis, amytal), and given a positive outlook for function. The child must also be given insight into the reason for his symptoms. If his symptoms are so disabling, i.e., convulsions, coma, paralysis, etc., his school is to be contacted and encouraged to cooperate so that it too is mobilized to help the child cope and develop stronger defense mechanisms. Only through this environmental alteration can the child hope to achieve good results.

In cases where the parents are the precipitating influence in a disturbed parent-child relationship, the best therapy is separation and hospitalization. Individual psychological support is given to the patient and also to the parents in an attempt to correct the delicate balance. Only by enlightment and mutual respect can we hope to be successful. The importance of collaborative care with paramedical and medical personnel is an essential ingredient in patient management and success.

8

PSYCHODYNAMICS

Many controversial explanations have been offered to account for hysterical conversion reactions, yet for those of us involved in clinical medicine, one cannot deny its existence. There are some who claim that there is no such condition and others who explain it as a normal response to stress. Other theories claim that hysterical conversion reactions indicate a primary psychiatric disease, such as schizophrenia, recurrent depression or character disorder, which is preceded by hysterical symptoms. Others account for hysteria as forerunners of neurological disease. Despite the fact that the proponents for each of these theories quote from specific literature, it becomes obvious, upon review of these studies, that they are inaccurate in the choice of studies and the relevant etiological factors.

At first glance, it is difficult to grasp how such physical symptoms as pain, blindness or paralysis, may, in fact, be expressing ideas or fantasies, rather than be the result of bodily changes. The most widely accepted theory is that proposed by Freud, whose theory holds that the hysterical personality structure develops at the genital level and is due to a failure in the resolution of the Oedipal conflict. According to Freudian theory, hysterical symptoms are disguised memory traces of sexual traumata (real and imagined) which have been repressed in childhood; this repression has failed however in later life. The development of the symptoms is an attempt to resolve the psychological conflict. If the resolution is unsuccessful, anxiety is reduced and the patient achieves a "*primary gain*". Thus, the patient may appear little concerned about the symptoms and demonstrate *la belle indifference*, despite words to the contrary. In addition to reducing anxiety, which is an intra-psychic process, the conversion symptom further serves to help cope with a threatening environment by removing the patient from situations that are potentially a threat. This is known as "*secondary gain.*" Clinical experience reveals that the majority of adult patients have sexual conflicts, but other personality conflicts are also seen during detailed psychiatric interviews and on psychological testing. There is always a *purposive aspect* to these hysterical conversion reactions, whether they occur during wartime, periods of danger, prison or an injury of related compensation. We physicians tend to view illness as being "bad" by dint of our extensive training, but we tend to forget that illness also can have positive aspects that can far outweigh the negative. This is especially true during wartime, for example in Viet Nam, where soldiers intentionally wounded themselves to avoid or evade dangerous assignments. Thus, the total relationship between the body and the mind remains complex, multifaceted and difficult to penetrate. We must consider these reactions as a form of non-verbal communication and if we understand the specific body language, we can deal more effectively with them from a therapeutic standpoint.

9

MANAGEMENT

After the neurological examination has confirmed that the symptoms represent hysterical conversion reactions, the psychological makeup of the patient should be probed so that the physician may have insight into the symptoms and their possible causes. A family tree of medical illness and a time flow chart of life events and medical care constructed by the physician will serve as a useful guide. Since life events and stress precipitate conversion reactions, the clinician must have a firm understanding of the patient's ego strengths and also understand how they have previously reacted to stressful situations. Family dynamics are also of extreme importance, not only in the acute precipitation of symptoms, but also in the therapeutic area. This history usually requires several sessions. When it is complete, the physician will be able to appreciate the patient's ego strengths, how he reacts to stress and daily living experiences, and specifically, the acute emotional stress that precipitated the hysterical conversion reaction. The patient experiences the deficits as real and rejects the fact that the symptoms are psychological. The physician must consider the patient just as impaired, as if the symptoms were organic in origin. It is important for the physician to be sensitive to the needs of the patient and not to respond with hostility. This is an art one cultivates, not a technique one learns. Unfortunately, many physicians do not appreciate this and demonstrate disdain for the patient by performing demeaning indignities, such as placing a surgical clamp on "an anesthetic breast." The physician may also give up on the patient as not worth the effort because he or she is obviously faking. This reaction by the physician is usually subconscious and is basically a response to the frustrating and hostility-provoking behavior of many patients. Thus, the physician's negative emotional reaction to his patient can overwhelm his diagnostic abilities even when sufficient information is available. Recent articles have confirmed how physicians' attitudes can vary under different circumstances and toward the different sexes. These attitudes and practices do not necessarily parallel scientific literature or recommendations. Some novice physicians curtly tell their patients that the symptoms are all in their minds. Invariably, the patients' conditions deteriorate, new symptoms may develop and the patients are unable to work out their emotional problems. Since these hysterical conversion reactions have a protective value for the patient, they must be dealt with respectfully and cautiously until the symbolism becomes obvious. In many cases, the precipitating event is relatively simple to understand.

If a patient appears to be a reasonably stable individual with a strong personality, then supportive treatment by the general practitioner, internist, and neurologist is appropriate. The removal of the symptoms is then generally achieved with little difficulty. However, it must be stressed that this is the first part of the treatment process. Suggestion, placebo, sodium amytal or hypnosis are all effective.

Hafeiz describes his experience in 61 patients using the method of suggestion with four specific procedures:

1. Faradic stimulation — briefly applied to involved limbs.
2. Somlec: an electro-sleeping machine that primarily produces relaxation. It is applied to the head for 30–60 minutes, while suggestion is carried out.
3. Sodium amytal — 250 mg in 5 ml given IV at rate of 1 ml/min.
4. Methylamphetamine — 10 mg IV.

He randomly allocated patients to one of these procedures. He informed each patient that his symptom was considered serious and that it would disappear after treatment. While the treatment was in progress, the patient was informed by suggestion that the symptom was disappearing. He was encouraged to practice the lost function until full recovery was achieved. One method was repeated three to four times before another was undertaken. Hafeiz was impressed that the removal of the symptom was usually accompanied by emotionally charged scenes of sighing, tears or shaking. The response to suggestion under faradic stimulation was best at 90% and Somlec at 84%. Methedrine injections produced 81% benefit, whereas sodium amytal only 20%. The latter procedure was ultimately abandoned. His experience with response of specific types of symptoms to this modality is similar to my own, in that patients with gross motor paralyses, tremor and aphonia respond better than those with hysterical convulsions or chronic pain.

If the patient is emotionally complex, it is advisable to obtain the aid of a competent psychiatrist, with the patient's permission. It is extremely important that the conversion not be removed unless the clinician is ready to offer aggressive psychological supportive treatment to determine the etiology. If this aspect is neglected, it sets up the patient for a chronic and disabling illness. According to Steinhart, the approach to treatment must be individualized. Although the emphasis is on rapid treatment to prevent the reinforcement of secondary gain and to avoid chronic disability, he correctly emphasizes the need to remove these symptoms with respect and not by deception. In general, there are two types of treatment for conversion hysteria. Those which are symptom-oriented with emphasis on return to function and those which deal with the total personality. As a rule, both approaches should allow for the patient to gently be exposed to the possibility that emotional factors are causative. Treatment must be tailored to the individual patient. In reviewing and evaluating the effectiveness of psychotherapy, one must be circumspect as to the claims made. It is clear that spontaneous symptomatic recovery occurs and is fairly common as soon as the external precipitating event is removed from the environment. It is of interest to note that 60% of Ljungberg's cases and 75% of Carter's patients recovered within one to five years. With these cases, it was usually possible to clearly identify a significant precipitating event. The event was often transient and unlikely to be re-experienced soon. Under such circumstances, when the precipitating event passed and the emotional intensity attached to it dissipated with the passage of time, the majority of patients recovered. However, in attempting to determine prognosis, the specific choice and duration of therapy rests not on the nature of the presenting symptoms, but rather on the patient's underlying personality structure. Hafeiz found his relapse rate was low and significantly related to the duration of symptoms before treatment. The longer a symptom is present the greater chance for relapse. Long term psychoanalysis attempts to give the patient insight into the problem and helps to reshape the ego defense posture.

Psychological tests may be helpful but alone they never establish the diagnosis. There are several tests that are routinely used but three specific batteries offer the most information. The Rorschach Test and Thematic Aperception Test (TAT) are projective tests that often provide rich, dynamic material, especially in children. These can give the clinician insight into the associations, imagery, preoccupations, conflicts and defense mechanisms of the individual. The Minnesota Multiphasic Personality Inventory (MMPI) has several scales of which the hypochondriasis (HS) and hysteria (HY) are more consistently answered. Serial analysis of drawing of a figure may be helpful in determining maturation of body concepts.

The physician and psychiatrist who find that the hysterical conversion reactions are persisting and protracted must diligently search for an organic etiology or consider the patient to be a schizophrenic. The high incidence of organic pathology, as noted by Slater, should emphasize that the diagnosis of hysterical conversion reaction must be made on positive evidence rather than as a diagnosis of exclusion. It can be hazardous for both the patient and the physician if these rules are not followed. Symptoms associated with organic disease often reflect exaggerations of basic personality or regression to earlier coping behavior. It is imperative for physicians to remain alert when caring for patients with hysterical conversion reaction despite the fact that organic aspects are not present. There is always a danger when using the term, "hysteria" and "hysterical conversion reaction," in that it tends to close the physician's eyes to organicity.

An interesting report by Tissenbaum and workers reviewed 395 neurological cases and reported that 53 (13.4%) had been called "functional" for varying periods ranging from one to eight years before the correct neurological diagnosis. Within four years after initial evaluation, 33 of the 53 "functional" patients (62%) had been found to have organic disease of the nervous system. It is clear that serial evaluation of these patients will help clarify some of the complexities. The contribution of organic disease to hysterical phenomenon is substantial and, consequently, the physician must remain vigilant. Lewis, Slater, Merskey, Whitlock and Weintraub have emphasized this association to the point where the traditional compartmentalization of medical/surgical (organic) and psychiatric syndrome becomes dangerous because the usual rules of diagnosis of organicity are suspended by a "label." This label ultimately may lead to inadequate diagnosis and improper treatment. Whitlock feels that the reticular activating system is altered producing the organic component of HCR. Thus there is some support for the claim that particular cerebral organic diseases may predispose to the development of HCR.

Clinical experience has shown that functional overreaction to organic disease as demonstrated by examination techniques is not uncommon. The diagnosis of one does not invalidate the diagnosis of the other and each will probably blur the other's presentation. Absolute statistics are difficult to obtain on this occurrence. The combination of hysteria and multiple sclerosis serves as a model for the co-existence of organic and psychological disorders. An excellent review of this association was recently published by Caplan and Nadelson demonstrating how the sick deal with their infirmities and how the physician comprehensively deals with illness. They emphasize that there is a continuum of responses of the organism ranging from the purely affective through symptoms of disease to disease states in response to psychological and physical stresses in the environment. In addition, these authors believe that it is necessary to recognize that neurological disability exists in the context of life's demands rather than to view a disease as an isolated phenomenon.

It is clear that diagnostic shortcomings in the past were responsible for the low rate of discovery of organic lesions. In this new era of CAT, NMR, PET etc., the neurologist will be able to identify and categorize patients accurately and can more effectively manage these individuals. Accurate statistical data can then be generated and thereby help clear up some of the confusion regarding hysterical illness.

CONCLUSIONS

Although HCR is not readily suited to direct experimentation, it is clear that a new approach is necessary if we are to understand the contemporary hysteric. As a term, hysteria has been used indiscriminately and interchangeably to the point where it has become a subterfuge for ignorance. Too great a reliance on personality, diagnosis by exclusion and opinions and observations only of psychiatrists has led to a distorted and confused picture of this entity. This monograph is an attempt to place the entity of HCR under strict guidelines, with diagnosis only by *positive* findings. By emphasizing this cautious, yet comprehensive approach, precise statistical data can be generated. It would be a mistake to assume that HCR are a phenomena in isolation. Clearly this phenomena may occur in any person at any point in time, yet there is a clear-cut predilection for women. With the introduction of the highly accurate CAT scan and the emergence of nuclear magnetic resonance (NMR) and PET, reliable data will be developed. The coexistence of organic and functional disease and the role of the distorted symbolic communication with its primary and secondary gains will be further explored.

I do not believe any useful purpose is served by removing the term hysteria and replacing it with "Briquet's Syndrome" or "psychogenic sensory-motor disturbance" because the term is so firmly entrenched. However, we as physicians must become more specific and accurate when applying this term. Many physicians still think of HCR in terms of the dramatic presentations of Charcot but contemporary HCR have become somewhat more subtle with frequent presentations of pain, headache and unexplained disability. Clearly the primary care physicians and neurologists must assume a more prominent role if we are ever to obtain accurate data and understand the role that emotions play.

Thus hysteria remains one of the most difficult and dangerous diagnoses in contemporary medicine. It is shrouded in controversy yet exists as a common clinical problem and thereby imposes unique demands on the clinician. Positive evidence must exist to accurately establish the diagnosis. Successful management requires the rare combination of a knowledge of neuroanatomy, psychiatric skills, experience, compassion and understanding.

REFERENCES

Abse, D.W. *Hysteria and Related Mental Disorders*. William and Wilkins, Baltimore, Maryland, 1966.

Akhtar, S., Brenner, I. "Differential Diagnosis of Fugue-Like States," *Journal Clinical Psych* 40:381–385, 1979.

Aldrich, C.K., *Psychiatry for the Family Physician*. Blakiston Division, McGraw-Hill, New York, 1954.

Apley, J., "The Child with Abdominal Pains," *Blackwell Scientific Publications*. Oxford, England, 1959.

Arkonac, O. and Guze, S.B., "A Family Study of Hysteria," *New England Journal of Medicine*, 268:238–242, 1963.

Barr, R.G., Levine, D.L., Watkins, J.B., "Lactose Malabsorption Has a Substantial Role in the Symptoms of Children with Recurrent Abdominal Pain," *New England Journal of Medicine*, 300:1448–1452, 1979.

Bastian, H.C., *Paralyses: Cerebral, Bulbar and Spinal*. Lewis, London, 1886.

Berger, D.M., "Hysteria: In Search of the Animus," *Comp. Psych.* 12:277–286, 1971.

Berney, T.P., "A Review of Simulated Illness," *South African Medical Journal*, 47:1429–1434, 1973.

Bibb, R.C. and Guze, S.B., "Hysteria (Briquet's Syndrome) in a Psychiatric Hospital," *American Journal of Psychiatry* 129:224–228, 1972.

Binnie, C.D., Rowan, A.J., Overweg, J. et al., "Telemetric EEG and Video Monitoring in Epilepsy," *Neurology* 31:298–303, 1981.

Breuer, J. and Freud, S., "Studies on Hysteria," in Standard Edition of *The Complete Works of Sigmund Freud*, Volume II, Hogarth Press, London, 1955.

Boweby, J., *Personality and Mental Illness*. Emerson Brooks, New York, 1942.

Briquet, P., *Traité Clinque et Therapeutique à l'Hysterie*, J.B. Balliere and Fils, Paris, 1859.

Bursten, B., "Munchausen's Syndrome," *Arch. Gen. Psych.* 13:261–268, 1965.

Carden, N.L., Schramel, D.J., "Observations of Conversion Reactions Seen in Troops Involved in the Viet Nam Conflict," *American Journal Psych.*, 123:21–31, 1966.

Carter, A.B., "The Prognosis of Certain Hysterical Symptoms," *British Medical Journal*, 1:1076–1079, 1949.

Chambers, W.R., "Neurological Conditions Masquerading as Psychiatric Diseases," *American Journal Psych.*, 112:387–389, 1955.

Chenven, M.S., Use of Children's Drawings as Diagnostic Aids. Presented at Meeting American Academy of Child Psychiatry, October, 1978, San Diego, California.

Chodoff, P. and Lyons, H., "Hysteria, The Hysterical Personality and 'Hysterical' Conversion," *American Journal Psych.*, 114:734–740, 1958.
Cleghorn, R.A., "Hysteria — Multiple Manifestations of Semantic Confusion," *Can. Psych. Assoc. J.*, 14:539–551, 1969.
Cohen, M.E., Robins, E., Purtell, J.J., et al., "Excessive Surgery in Hysteria. Study of Surgical Procedures in Fifty Women with Hysteria and One Hundred Ninety Controls," *JAMA*, 151:977–986, 1953.
Cohen, R.J., Suter, C., "Hysterical Seizures—The Use of Saline Infusion and Suggestion as a Provocative Test in Forty-one Cases," *Annals Neurology*, 8:98, 1980.
Crawford, J.P., "Hysteria and Schizophrenia," *Lancet*, 2:269–270, 1979.
Currie, S., Heathfield, K.W.G., Henson, R.A., et al., "Clinical Course and Prognosis of Temporal Lobe Epilepsy — A Survey of 666 Patients," *Brain*, 94:173–190, 1971.
Cusamano, J.V., Fletcher, J.W., Patel, B.K., "Scintigraphic Appearance of Anton's Syndrome," *JAMA*, 245:1248–1249, 1981.
Deutsch, F., *On the Mysterious Leap from the Mind to the Body*, International Universities Press, New York, 1959.
Devereaux, G., "Mohave Ethno-Psychiatry and Suicide: The Psychiatric Knowledge and the Psychic Disturbance of an Indian Tribe," Bureau of American Ethnology, Bulletin 175, 1961.
Diagnostic and Statistical Manual of Mental Disorders, Edition 2, Washington, D.C., American Psychiatric Association, 1968.
Diagnostic and Statistical Manual of Mental Disorders, Edition 3, Washington, D.C., American Psychiatric Association, 1978.
Desai, B.T., Porter, R.J., Penry, J.K., "The Psychogenic Seizure by Videotaped Analysis: A Study of 42 Attacks in Six Patients," *Neurology*, April, 1979, p. 602.
Drews, R.C., "Organic vs. Functional Ocular Problems," International Ophthalmological Clinic, 7:665–696, 1967.
Editorial: Thermography — Aches and Pains, February, 1981, p. 8–11.
Engel, G.L., " 'Psychogenic' Pain and the Pain-Prone Patient," *Amer. Journal of Medicine*, 26:899–918, 1959.
Ehrlich, E.L., Fisher, R.L., "Orthopedic Conversion Reactions in Children and Adolescents," *Conn. Med.*, 41:681–683, 1977.
Faigel, H.C., "The Wandering Womb: Mass Hysteria in Schoolgirls," *Clinical Ped.*, 7:377–378, 1968.
Farley, J., Woodruff, R.A., and Guze, S.B., "The Prevalence of Hysteria and Conversion Symptoms," *British Journal of Psychiatry*, 114:1121–1125, 1968.
Fenichel, O., *Conversion in the Psychoanalytic Theory of Neurosis*, Chapter 12, W.W. Norton, New York, 1945.
Fitzgerald, O.W.S., "Love Deprivation and the Hysterical Personality," *Journal Mental Science*, 94:701–717, 1948.
Flannery, R.B., Sos, J., McGovern, P., "Ethnicity as a Factor in the Expression of Pain" *Psychosomatics*, 22:39–50, 1981.
Flemenbaum, A., "Hysterical Neurosis — Conversion Type," *Minnesota Med.*, 55:853–857, 1972.
Forbis, O.L. and James, R.H., "Hysteria in Childhood," *Southern Medical Journal*, 58:1221–1225, 1965.

Forrester, R.M., "Epidemic Hysteria — Divide and Conquer," *British Medical Journal*, 669, September 15, 1979.
Freedman, A.M. and Kaplan, H.I., *Comprehensive Text Book of Psychiatry*, William and Wilkins, Baltimore, Md., 1967.
Friedman, A., Wood, E.H.: Thermography in Vascular Headache (Chap. 7) in Medical Thermography, Theory and Clinical Applications. Brentwood Publishing Corp., Los Angeles, California, 1976.
Freud, S., *Fragment of an Analysis of a Case of Hysteria*, Hogarth Press, London, 1955.
Friedman, S.B., "Conversion Symptoms in Adolescents," *Pediatric Clinics North America*, 20:873–882, 1973.
Fuente, J.R., Hanson, N.P., Duncan, G.M., et al., "A New Look at Ganser's Syndrome," *Psychiatric Annals*, 10:62–68, 1980.
Ganser, S.J., "Uber Einen Eigenartigen Hysterischen Dammerzustand," *Arch. F. Psych.*, Berlin, 30:633–640, 1898.
Gold, S., "Diagnosis and Management of Hysterical Contracture in Children," *British Medical Journal*, 5426:21–23, 1965.
Goodwin, J., Simms, M., Bergman, R., "Hysterical Seizures: A Sequel to Incest," *American Orthopsych. Assoc.*, 49:698–703, 1979.
Gross, M., "Pseudo Epilepsy: A Study of Adolescent Hysteria," *American Journal Psych.*, 136:210–213, 1979.
Gross, M.P. and Sloan, S.H., "Patients with Eye Symptoms and No Organic Illness: An Interdisciplinary Study," *Psych. Med.*, 2:298–307, 1971.
Gull, W.W., "Address in Medicine," *Lancet*, 2:171–176, 1868.
Gull, W.W., "Anorexia Hysterica (Apepsia Hysterica)," *British Medical Journal*, 2:527–528, 1873.
Gull, W.W., "Anorexia Nervosa (Apepsia Hysterica, Anorexia Hysterica)," *Trans. Clin. Soc.*, London, 7:22–28, 1874.
Guze, S.B., "The Diagnosis of Hysteria: What Are We Trying to Do?" *American Journal Psychiatry*, 124:491–497, 1967.
Guze, S.B., "The Role of Follow-Up Studies: Their Contribution to Diagnostic Classification as Applied to Hysteria," *Seminar Psych.* 2:392–402, 1970.
Guze, S.B., "Suicide, Hysteria and Conversion Symptoms," *JAMA*, 225:65, 1973.
Guze, S.B., and Perley, M.J., "Observations on the Natural History of Hysteria," *American Journal Psychiatry*, 119:960–965, 1963.
Hafeiz, H.B., "Hysterical Conversion: A Prognostic Study," *British Journal Psych.*, 136:548–551, 1980.
Hammer, H.M., "Astasia-Abasia: A Report of Two Cases at West Point," *Amer. J. Psych.*, 124:671–674, 1967.
Hammer, H.M., "Psychogenic Pain," *Journal Medical Society, New Jersey*, 70:757–759, 1973.
Hart, H.H., "The Eye in Symbol and Symptom," *The Psychoanalytical Review*, 36:1–21, 1949.
Head, H., "The Diagnosis of Hysteria," *British Medical Journal*, 1:827–829, 1922.
Hendler, N., Viernstein, M., et al.: A preoperative screening test for chronic back pain patients. Psychosomatics, 20:801–808, 1979.

Hillard, J.R., Rockwell, W.J.K., "Dysesthesias, Witchcraft and Conversion Reactions," *JAMA*, 240:1742–1744, 1978.
Janet, P., *The Major Symptoms of Hysteria, Second Edition*, MacMillan, New York, 1920.
Jensen, S.E., "The Indications for Abdominal Surgery in Psychiatric Patients, *Can. Psych. Assoc. J.*, 8:267–271, 1963.
Jones, A.B. and Llewllyn, L.J., *Malingering on the Simulation of Disease*, P. Blaketon & Son, Philadelphia, 1917.
Kalman, T.P., Granet, R.B., "The Written Interview in Hysterical Mutism," *Psychosomatics*, 22:362–366, 1981.
Kanner, L., *Child Psychiatry*, Third Edition, Charles E. Thomas, Springfield.
Keane, J.R., "Neuro-ophthalmic Signs and Symptoms of Hysteria," *Neurology*, 32:757–762, 1982.
Kennedy, A., and Neville, J., "Sudden Loss of Memory," *British Medical Journal*, 2:428–433, 1957.
Keschner, M., "Simulation of Nervous and Mental Disease," *Michigan Law Review*, 44:715–774, 1946.
Knight, J.A., Friedman, T.I., Sulianti, J., "Epidemic Hysteria: A Field Study," *American Journal Public Health*, 55:858–864, 1965.
Kretschmer, E., *Hysteria, Nervous and Mental Disease*, Publishing Company, New York, 1926.
Kruger, D.W., "Unilateral Ptosis as a Conversion Reaction," *Journal of Clin. Psych.*, April, 1978, pp. 351–356.
LaBarbera, J.D., Dozier, J.E., "Hysterical Seizures: The Role of Sexual Exploitation," *Psychosomatics*, 21:897–903, 1980.
Lader, M. and Sartorius, N., "Anxiety in Patients with Hysterical Conversion Symptoms," *Journal Neurol., Neurosurg., Psychiat.*, 31:490–495, 1968.
Laidlaw, J., Rickens, A., *A Textbook of Epilepsy*, Churchill and Livingtston, New York, pp. 160–161, 1976.
Langness, L.L., "Hysterical Psychosis: The Cross-Cultural Evidence," *American Journal Psychiatry*, 124:47–56, 1967.
Lapido, O.A., "Pseudocyesis in Infertile Patients," *Int. J. Gynaecol. Obstet.*, 16:427–429, 1979.
Laughlin, H.P., "The Conversion Reactions," Med. Ann. D.C., 22:581–594, 1953.
Lerner, M.A., "Hysterical Abdominal Proptosis," *American Journal Roentgenol, Radium, Ther. Nucl. Med.*, 122:275–277, 1974.
Lesser, R.P., Fahn, S., "Dystonia: A Disorder Often Misdiagnosed as a Conversion," *American Journal Psych.*, 135:349–352, 1978.
Lester, D., "Hysteria and Suicide," *JAMA*, 224:902, 1973.
Levine, R.J., "Epidemic Faintness and Syncope in a School Marching Band," *JAMA*, 238:2373–2376, 1977.
Levine, R.J., Sexton, D.J., et al., "Outbreak of Psychosomatic Illness at a Rural Elementary School," *Lancet* 2:1500–1503, 1974.
Lewis, W.C., "Hysteria: The Consultants' Dilemma," *Archives General Psych.*, 30:145–151, 1974.

Lewis, W.C. and Berman, M., "Studies of Conversion Hysteria," *Archives General Psych.*, 13:275–282, 1965.
Linton, R., *Culture and Mental Disorders*, Springfield, Illinois, Charles C. Thomas, 1956.
Ljungberg, L., "Hysteria — A Clinical, Prognostic and Genetic Study," *Acta. Psych. and Neuro Scand. Suppl.*, Volume 112, 1957.
Lucas, A.R., "Toward the Understanding of Anorexia Nervosa as a Disease Entity," Mayo Clinic Proceedings, 56:254–264, 1981.
Luisada, P.V., Peele, R. and Pittard, E.A., "The Hysterical Personality in Men," *American Journal Psych.*, 131:518–522, 1974.
Malmquist, C.P., "Hysteria in Childhood," *Post-Grad. Medicine*, 50:112–117, 1971.
Maloney, M.J., "Diagnosing Hysterical Conversion Reactions in Children," *J. Ped.*, 97:1016–1020, 1980.
Marmor, J., "Orality in the Hysterical Personality," *Journal Amer. Psychoanalytical Assoc.*, 1:656, 671, 1953.
Martin, R.L., Roberts, W.V., Clayton, P.J., "Psychiatric Status after Hysterectomy," *JAMA*, 244:350–353, 1980.
McGooty, V. Benhart, 305 Ill. APP 458 27 N.E. (Second) 289, 1940.
McKegney, F.P., "Auditory Hallucinations as a Conversion Symptom," *Comp. Psych.*, 8:80–89, 1967.
McKell, T.E., Sullivan, A.J., "The Hyperventilation Syndrome in Gastroenterology," *Gastroenterology*, 9:6–10, 1947.
Meloff, K.L., DeMeuron, G., Buncic, J.R., "Conversion Sixth-Nerve Palsy in a Child," *Psychosomatics*, 21:769–770, 1980.
Merskey, H., Buhrich, N.A., "Hysteria and Organic Brain Disease," *British Journal Med. Psychol.*, 48:359–366, 1975.
Mesulam, M.M., "Dissociative States with Abnormal Temporal Lobe EEG," *Arch. Neur.*, 38:176–181, 1981.
Miller, F., Korsvik, H., "Baclofen in the Treatment of Stiff Man Syndrome," *Ann. Neurol.*, 9:511–512, 1981.
Miller, H. and Cartlidge, N., "Simulation and Malingering After Injuries to the Brain and Spinal Cord," *Lancet*, 1:580–585, 1972.
Mucha, T.F. and Reinhardt, R.F., "Conversion Reactions in Student Aviators," *American Journal Psych.*, 127:493–497, 1970.
Nemiah, J.C., "Conversion: Fact or Chimera?" *International Journal Psychiatry Medicine*, 5:443–448, 1974.
New York Times, October 21, 1980, Section C-3. "Heat 'Pictures' of Pain Expected to Aid Sufferers, Detect Fakers."
Noble, D., "Hysterical Manifestations in Schizophrenic Illness," *Psych.*, 14:153–160, 1951.
Noyes, A.P. and Kolb, L.C., *Modern Clinical Psychiatry*, 6th Edition, W.S. Saunders, Philadelphia, 1963.
Ossipox, V.P., "Malingering: A Simulation of Psychosis," Bull Menninger, 8:39–42, 1944.
Page, H., *Injuries of the Spine and Spinal Cord Without Apparent Mechanical*

Lesions and Nervous Shock, London, Churchill, 1882.

Perley, M.J. and Guze, S.B., "Hysteria, The Stability and Usefulness of Clinical Criteria," *New England Journal of Medicine*, 266:421–426, 1962.

Pincus, J.H., Tucker, G.J., *Behavioral Neurology*, Oxford University Press, 1978.

Plum, F., Posner, J.B., *Diagnosis of Stupor in Coma*, F. A. Davis Company, 1966.

Proctor, J.F., "The Treatment of Hysteria in Childhood" in Hammer, M. and Kaplan, A.M. edition, *The Practice of Psychotherapy with Children*, Dorsey Press, Homeward, Illinois, 1967.

Purtell, J.J., Robins, E. and Cohen, M.E., "Observations on Clinical Aspects of Hysteria," — a quantitative study of 50 hysteria patients and 156 controlled subjects, *JAMA*, 146:902–909, 1951.

Putnam, J.J., "Recent Investigation into the Pathology of So-called Concussion of the Spine," *Boston Medical and Surgical Journal*, 109:217–220, 1883.

Rada, R.T., Meyer, G.G. and Krill, A.E., "Visual Conversion Reactions in Children," *Psychosomatics*, 10:23–28, 1969.

Rice, D.G. and Greenfield, N.S., "Psychophysiological Correlates of LaBelle Indifférence," *Archives General Psychiatry*, 20:239–245, 1969.

Riley, T., Massey, D.W., "Pseudoseizures vs. Real," *Emergency Medicine*, 11:122–129, 1979.

Robins, E. and O'Neal, P., "Clinical Features of Hysteria with a Note on Prognosis," *Nerv Child*, 10:246–271, 1953.

Rosenthal, R.H., Webb, W.L. and Wruble, L.D., "Diagnosis and Management of Persistent Psychogenic Vomiting," *Psychosomatics*, 21:722–730, 1980.

Sackellares, J.C., Giordani, B., Boll, T.J., et al., "Neuropsychological Performances of Patients with Pseudoseizures," *Epilepsia*, 22:244, 1981.

Schatzki, R.P., "Globus Hystericus (Globus Sensation)," *New England Journal of Medicine*, 270:676, 1964.

Schneider, S., Rice, D.R., "Neurologic Manifestations of Childhood Hysteria," *Journal Pediatrics*, 94:153–156, 1979.

Seitz, P.F.D., "Experiments in the Substitution of Symptoms by Hypnosis," *Psychosomatic Medicine*, 15:405–424, 1953.

Shaw, R.S., "Pathologic Malingering. The Painful Disabled Extremities," *New England Journal Medicine*, 271:22–26, 1964.

Simelpoulos, A.M. and Reissman, H.H., "Progressive Hysterical Tetraplegia with Contractures, A Case Study," *John Hopkins Medical Journal*, 125:14–18, 1969.

Slater, E., "Diagnosis of Hysteria," *British Medical Journal*, 1:1395–1399, 1965.

Slater, E., and Glithero, E., "A Follow-Up of Patients Diagnosed as Suffering from 'Hysteria'," *Journal Psychosomatic Research*, 9:9–13, 1965.

Sperling, M., "Conversion Hysteria and Conversion Symptoms: And Revision of Classification and Concepts," *Journal American Psychoanalytic Assoc.*, 21:745–771, 1973.

Standage, K.F., "The Etiology of Hysterical Seizures," *Canadian Psychiatric Assoc. Journal*, 20:67–73, 1975.

Steffinis, C., Markidis, M., and Christodoulou, G., "Observations on the

Evolution of the Hysterical Symptomatology," *British Journal Psychiatry*, 128:269–275, 1976.
Stephens, J.H. and Kamp, M., "On Some Aspects of Hysteria: A Clinical Study," Journal Nervous Mental Disease, 134:305–315, 1962.
Stevens, H., "Conversion Hysteria, A Neurologic Emergency," *Mayo Clinic Proceedings*, 43:54–64, 1968.
Stewart, S.G., Randall, G.C., and Riesenman, F.R., "Hysterical Homonomous Hemianopsia with Hemiplegia," *War Medicine*, 40:606–607, 1943.
Sydenham, T., "Epistolatory Dissertation to Dr. Cole In: The Works of Thomas Sydenham," Vol. 2:85–118, Sydenham Soc., London, 1850.
Tissenbaum, M.J., Harter, H.M. and Friedman, A.P., "Organic Neurological Syndrome Diagnoses as Functional Disorders," *JAMA*, 147:1519–1521, 1951.
Troost, B.T. and Troost, E.G., "Functional Paralysis of Horizontal Gaze," *Neurology*, 29:82–85, 1979.
Ulett, P.C. and Gildea, E.F., "Survey of Surgical Procedures In Psychoneurotic Women," *JAMA*, 143:960–963, 1950.
Veith, I., *Hysteria, the History of a Disease*, University of Chicago Press, Chicago, 1965.
Ventry, I.M., "Bekesy Audiometry in Functional Hearing Loss: A Case Study," *Journal of Speech and Hearing Disorders*, 36:125–141, 1971.
Waggoner, R.V., Bagchi, B.K., "Initial Masking of Organic Brain Changes by Psychic Symptoms," *American Journal Psychiatry*, 110:904–910, 1954.
Wallace, C.M., "Looking at Psychiatry. Nursing the Hysterical Patient," *Nursing Mirror*, 136:10–41, 1973.
Waller, D.A., "Paroxysmal Kinesigenic Choreathetosis or Hysteria?" *American Journal Psychiatry*, 134:1439–1440, 1977.
Walshe, F.M.R., "Diagnosis of Hysteria," *British Medical Journal*, 2:1451–1454, 1965.
Walshe, F.M.R., *Diseases of the Nervous System*, Williams and Wilkins, Baltimore, 1963.
Walters, A., "The Psychogenic Regional Pain Syndrome (Hysterical Pain)," *Compre. Ther.*, 1:20–25, 1975.
Wechsler, I.S.A., *A Textbook of Clinical Neurology*, Saunders, Philadelphia, 1947.
Weinstein, E.A., Eck, R.A. and Lyerly, O.G., "Conversion Hysteria in Appalachia," *Psych.*, 32:334–341, 1969.
Weintraub, M.I., "Hysteria," *American Family Physician*, 8:91–95, 1973.
Weintraub, M.I., "Hysteria: A Clinical Guide to Diagnosis," (Monograph), *Clinical Symposia*, Vol. 29, pp. 1–30, Nov. 1977.
Weintraub, M.I., "A Clinician's Manual of Hysterical Conversion Reactions," Interdisciplinary Communications Media, 1978.
Weintraub, M.I., "How to Approach the Hysterical Patient," *Medical Times*, 110:50–54, Nov. 1982.
Werlin, S.L., D'Souza, B.J., et al., "Sandifer's Syndrome: An Unappreciated Clinical Entity," *Developmental Medicine and Child Neurology*, 22:374–378, 1980.

Whitlock, F.A., "The Aetiology of Hysteria," ACTA Psychiat. Scand. 43:144–162, 1967.

Woodruff, R.A., Clayton, P.J., and Guze, S.B., "Hysteria: An Evaluation of Specific Diagnostic Criteria by the Study of Randomly selected Psychiatric Clinic Patients," *British Journal Psych.*, 115:1243–1248, 1969.

Yasuna, E.R., "Hysterical Amblyopia in Children," *American Journal Disease of Childhood*, 106:558–564, 1963.

Yates, A. and Steward, M., "Conversion Hysteria in Childhood, A Case Report and a Reminder," *Clinical Pediatrics*, 15:379–382, 1976.

Ziegler, D.K. and Paul, N., "On the Natural History of Hysteria in Women" (A followup study twenty years after hospitalization), *Disease Nervous System*, 15:301–306, 1954.

Ziegler, F.J., "Hysterical Conversion Reactions," *Post Grad Med.*, 47:174–178, 1970.

Ziegler, F., Imboden, J. and Meyer, E., "Contemporary Conversion Reaction: A Clinical Study," *American Journal of Psychiatry*, 116:901–909, 1960.

Ziegler, F., Imboden, J., and Meyer, E., "Contemporary Conversion Reactions II: A Conceptual Model," *Arch. Gen. Psych.*, 6:279–286, 1962.

Ziegler, F., Imboden, J. and Rodgers, D.A., "Contemporary Conversion Reactions III, Diagnostic Considerations," *JAMA*, 186:307–311, 1963.

APPENDIX

APPENDIX: Tests

DESCRIPTION	ORGANIC LESION	HYSTERICAL LESION
A. Loss of smell 1. Patient closes eyes 2. Place familiar substances under nostrils 3. Place spirits of ammonia under nostrils	Patient unable to appreciate familiar substances (I) but able to perceive irritating ammonia (V)	No appreciation of all substances
B. Unilateral loss of vision The eye is examined for local causes of disease. The pupillary response to light is noted. The Marcus-Gunn pupillary test is performed by having patient fixate at distance in darkened room. A bright light is rapidly moved back-forth and stimulates both pupils. After a few seconds of light movement, the light is maintained on the affected eye. This is repeated on other eye.	Pupil constricts and remains constricted on normal eye. The pupil constricts initially and then dilates or springs larger indicating optic nerve disease.	Both pupils remain constricted
C. Bilateral loss of vision Examine eye for intrinsic disease. Test response to opto-kinetic drum (OKN) Determine if there is a response to threat. Determine if patient avoids obstacles in his path. Determine integrity of occipital lobes by photic driving response during electroencephalography (EEG)	Unable to follow OKN. No response to threat. Falls and trips over objects. No driving response to photic stimulation.	Responds to OKN & threat. Avoids danger. Normal PS response
D. Red Glass Test for unilateral blindness The patient is asked to read a line of alternating black and red letters (ABCDEFGH). A red glass is placed before "Normal" eye. (Note: Red letters are invisible when viewed through a red glass)	A C E G	ABCDEFGH

E. Lens test for unilateral blindness Examine eyes Place strong convex lens over "Normal" eye re-test acuity	Poor acuity	Normal acuity
F. Test for tunnel vision Test visual field at 10 feet. Test visual field at 20 or 30 feet.	Larger visual field	No change
G. Monocular diplopia testing. Examine eyes to rule out intrinsic disease or paresis. 1. Use red-green glass testing to determine peripheral image; repeat several times and reverse colors. 2. Use prisms (Neg and Pos) over good eye to determine vision in "bad" eye.	(1) Usually find dislocated lens or intrinsic eye pathology.	(1) Changing pattern (No consistency) (2) Vision normal in "bad" eye
H. Unequal pupils (aniscoria) 1. Normal 2. Adie's pupil 3. Horner's sympathetic pupil 4. Argyll-Robertson pupil of Lues 5. Iatrogenic use of Homatropine (dilated and fixed pupil)	No change with drugs Sensitive to 2½% Mecholyl (constricts) Sensitive to 1:1000 adrenalin (constricts) No change with drugs No response to pilocarpine	
I. Test for deafness 1. Perform standard audiometric tests 2. Startle while asleep with loud sound 3. Look for K-complex during sleep EEG	May find sensory-neural changes Minimal to absent response Minimal to absent response	Normal Awakes & startled K-complex is well formed
J. Test for selective loss of speech volume Examine mouth, tongue and larynx. Ask patient to cough.	Abnormal Loud bovine cough (unable to approximate vocal cords)	Normal Loud normal cough
K. Sensory alteration (hemisensory, islands, etc.) Use pin, touch, position and vibration over dorsal and ventral portions of body	Hemisensory-decreased sensation over dorsal & ventral body with paramedian sparing	Absent Usually over front of body Sharp midline cutoff Changes on repeat testing

DESCRIPTION	ORGANIC LESION	HYSTERICAL LESION
1. Use pin, touch, position and vibration over dorsal and ventral portions of body 2. splitting of vibration over skull, sternum, ribs, etc.	Osteomyelitis or bone defect or tantalum plate	Normal bone
L. Test for extremity weakness or paralysis. (upper extr) 1. Patient supine and involved extremity (e.g., arm) is placed over patient's face and released. 2. Extremity placed in position of primary action of specific muscle. A sudden, unexpected, reverse pressure is exerted by examiner.	Hit face Can overcome strength	Falls safely to side Patient exhibits a strong counter response indicating reserve power.
M. Test of Leg weakness 1. Hoover test The patient is instructed to raise normal leg against resistance by examiner. Examiner's other hand is placed under "weak" heel to test for synergistic downthrust.	In true paralysis there is no synergistic downthrust	Good synergistic thrust is detected
2. Thigh adductor paralysis The examiner's hands are placed on both portions of the inner thigh. The patient is instructed to adduct the normal thigh against resistance of examiner. The other hand detects strength of the "weak" muscle	No synergistic contraction is detected	Good synergistic contraction detected
N. Test of coordination Patient closes eyes and is requested to place index finger on nose	Dysmetria	Smooth movement to other site, e.g., ear to eye

O. Test for gait abnormality. 1. Observe patient's gait. Determine if there is a fixed pattern to abnormality. Reverse their position.	Patient falls in a random manner. If previous stroke, will observe circumduction of leg. Look for classic gait alterations of Parkinson's disease, common peroneal palsy, peripheral neuropathy and cerebellar ataxia.	Patient always falls always to support. Will not hurt themselves.
P. Test for hysterical seizure 1. Observe activity and check for Babinski response, corneal reflex, and then place knuckles into sternum and press deeply.	In grand mal seizure there are tonic-clonic movements with loss of consciousness, bilateral Babinski, depressed corneal sensation. Minimal or no change to noxious stimulus.	There is no loss of consciousness, nor true tonic-clonic movements. No Babinski corneals are active if can test. Marked response to noxious stimulus by pushing examiner's hand or actually grabbing hand

Index

GPSR Compliance

The European Union's (EU) General Product Safety Regulation (GPSR) is a set of rules that requires consumer products to be safe and our obligations to ensure this.

If you have any concerns about our products, you can contact us on ProductSafety@springernature.com

In case Publisher is established outside the EU, the EU authorized representative is:

Springer Nature Customer Service Center GmbH
Europaplatz 3
69115 Heidelberg, Germany

Batch number: 10830943

Printed by Printforce, the Netherlands